THE LEAN

A Story to Give You the Motivation and Tools Needed for Lasting Fat Loss and Lifelong Health

By Brooks Hollan

www.fitlife212.com

July 2014
Copyright © 2011, 2014 Brooks Hollan
All rights reserved worldwide.

Published by Archangel Ink
ISBN: 1500447811
ISBN-13: 978-1500447816

The Lean Life

Acknowledgements

This book is dedicated to Heather in San Diego who got tired of being a passenger and decided to take control of her journey. She beat cancer, lost over 165 pounds, and has control over her life again. It all started with seemingly little steps--steps that really counted—and ended with her living The Lean Life.

The Lean Life is a story designed to inspire you, challenge you, and empower you to make small lifestyle changes that will pay big dividends in your journey called life. No matter where you are today, you can start taking little steps in the direction you want to go.

Thanks to all of my friends and family who supported me along the way in the creation of this book, but also in making The Lean Life a movement to empower millions of people to change their lives and the lives of their families for the better.

I would like to give a special 'thank you' to RWD for believing in the cause and for all of the timely input and suggestions.

I would like to give an extra special thanks to Drew Canole. This book would not have been possible without him in so many ways. It goes beyond his ideas and feedback that played a part in the creation of this book. Without his mentoring, support, and truly believing in me, I don't think I would have ever seen this through to completion. Drew is an amazing person, and I am lucky to call him a friend. Not to mention, I wouldn't have met Natalie if it weren't for Drew. Thanks for everything Drew, especially for believing in me.

Enjoy the book…

Brooks Hollan

The Lean Life

Foreword by Natalie Jill

The Lean Life is more than an enjoyable, heart-warming, and easy to read story about a family of five. It is an education about health and nutrition told through a story instead of a textbook 'do this, do that' format.

This story will bring you close to the life of a likeable kid named Timmy who finally had to confront his weight as he got older. Follow his journey as he goes off to college and meets a counselor and a trainer who turn his life around for the better.

I really liked his 'letters to mom' and how they seemed to do a great job of recapping what was learned. Plus, being a mom myself, I found them very touching!

You learn as Timmy learns, but more importantly, you will finish the book with a much greater understanding about the healthy nutritional habits that will make you yearn for more and ultimately set you on your way to a healthier, fitter future.

Even if you know about health, fitness, and nutrition; the way the book explains these concepts makes them simple and easy to understand. If you are a trainer or work with people, this aspect will help you better communicate with your clients as the explanations are great in this book!

The Lean Life concludes with a 22 page 'Fit Life workbook' that will help you fine-tune your life and your weight loss goals! As somebody with 20 years of experience in corporate goal setting and achievement, I really liked the simplicity of the program. In addition to the goals aspect, it gives you a simple yet solid nutritional plan that works and a KISS (Keep It Super Simple) handout with steps to get and keep you headed in the right direction!

I hope you enjoy your time with the Johnston family as much as I did.

-Natalie Jill

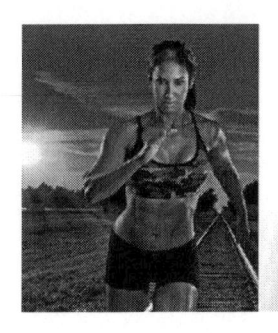

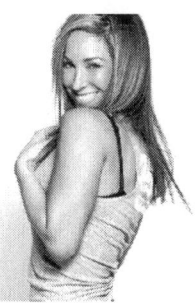

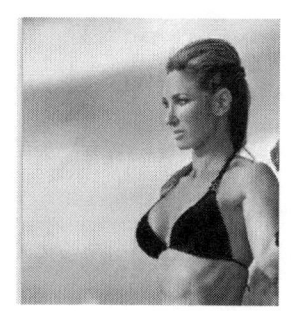

NatalieJillFitness.com

Natalie Jill Fitness

Table of Contents

Introduction	9
The Beginning	11
Eight Years Later	17
Then It Happened	20
On the Road	22
A Spark of Truth	26
On a Mission	30
In Search of Change	33
Letter to Mom #1	37
Timmy and the Trainer	39
Getting Bigger…Little by Little	44
America's Biggest Crisis – A Lack of Movement	49
Stop Lower Back Pain and Start Losing Weight	57
The Secret to Stopping Back Pain	66

	7
Just MOVE! A Little Goes a Long Way	75
Increase Your Metabolism by 3%	83
Salad Plates, Kiddie Bowls and Portion Control	90
Letter to Mom #2	97
See How You Want to Be	100
'Snooze' to Success	107
Affirmation Station	111
Letter to Mom #3	115
Motivation Strikes	118
No More Dieting	135
Starving Yourself Doesn't Work	141
Be a Fat-Burning Machine	151
Letter to Mom #4 – Speed Bumps and Recovery	161
How to Eat for Fat Loss	165
Let's Talk About Fat	174
Let's Talk About Carbs	179
Let's Talk About Protein	189
Putting It All Together – How to Build Your Meals	199
The Lean Life "KISS" Handout	201

The Lean Life "KISS" Handout	205
Vitamins	213
Don't Watch The Scale	216
Letter to Mom #5 – "Times are a Changing"	220
When Life Deals Lemons, Start Making Lemonade	223
Home for Thanksgiving	236
FitLife212 – Lifestyle Coaching: It's All About You	242
Lean Lifestyle Guide -"KISS" Handout	255
The Ten Commandments of a Lean Lifestyle	258
Food Journal	260
About the Author	261

The Lean Life

Introduction

Can you imagine a life for yourself or your loved ones with no more anguish and frustration over losing weight? Are you or somebody close to you tired of relying on self-control and deprivation in your unsuccessful attempts to lose weight?

If so, you are NOT alone. Whether you want to lose 10 pounds, 50 pounds, or even 100 pounds or more, there are tens of thousands of people that feel the exact same way you do.

You could be a child watching your parents get frustrated with yo-yo dieting. You could be an adult who is tired of wasting your time and money on weight loss gimmicks.

The good news is that you don't have to keep living this way.

By reading this book, you will see that you have an alternative to the dieting and frustration that comes with being or having a loved one that is overweight. With your busy lifestyle that revolves around job, kids, school, career, and/or family, there is often little time left to take care of one's health.

That is why creating a healthy lifestyle is so important. Creating good habits you will have for the rest of your life is the only thing that will work. The sooner you adopt these habits, the easier it will be for you to start living the life you want.

Most people don't learn or retain information very well when it is presented in a textbook format; they learn from the experiences of others, which are best told in the form of a story.

This book is designed to be entertaining and educational, and it is written in such a way that parents and children alike should read it. The sooner our children can adopt healthy lifestyle habits, the better off we will all become.

If you aren't battling weight issues yourself, great. I challenge you to be a positive impact on others. Everyone has a family member, friend, or co-worker that is battling weight issues; now is your time to step up to offer guidance and support.

Use this book as a tool to learn simple ways to explain and communicate with others. You can have all the right answers in the world, but if you can't communicate that to the people that need your help, it doesn't do much good.

If we work at it together, we can stop the obesity epidemic that is sweeping our country. If you take action to not only help yourself but also those you care about, we can reduce the increasing rates of childhood obesity, type-2 diabetes, and heart disease.

1

The Beginning

"Beep, Beep, Beep." It's 5:30 a.m. and the noise of the alarm clock shatters the early morning tranquility as Little Timmy reaches out from under the nest of covers and hits the snooze button. "Smack!"

The smell of homemade French toast with fresh maple syrup and pork sausage lingers throughout the beautiful antique farmhouse..

Timmy doesn't want to get out of bed; he knows that the first step on the cold hardwood floor will send a chill up the spine of his stocky 212-pound frame.

His mom, Susan, strides up the stairs to Timmy's second floor bedroom. He hears her footsteps, rolls over while pulling the covers up to his chin, and acts like he is still asleep. He lies there motionless, trying to squeeze out a couple more minutes of shut-eye before confronting the cold floor and another cruel day.

You see, I say "cruel" because Timmy is 212 pounds, but he's only 11 years old. You know how mean the other kids at school can be. Being picked on isn't as bad as always being picked last in PE class. It hurts worse because there is nowhere to hide and no way to avoid class.

Timmy often confided in his best friend Dan, who is skinny, that he was born this way. "Genetics," he would say. "It's normal because my whole family is this way. It's all I have ever known."

Enticed by the smell of French toast and sausage links, a smile crossed Timmy's face as he threw back the covers and attempted to roll out of bed. It took him a few seconds to sit up and move to the side of the bed; it's tough to move the extra weight around, especially on a big soft bed.

You wouldn't know his weight slowed him down by the way his feet danced on the cold floor and into the slippers he placed bedside every night.

With his feet protected, Timmy got dressed and headed downstairs to eat with his mom, dad, younger sister Jessica, and older brother Jason. Timmy was four years older than Jessica and six years younger than Jason.

Timmy saddled up to the large table like he owned the place. His nostrils were all set on French toast...that was until he saw Jason playing the latest edition Madden NFL video game on the 42-inch flat screen TV in the living room.

"Ha, ha, you just got intercepted," laughed Timmy.

"Jason, don't make me tell you again. Turn it off, NOW!" yelled Mom.

Timmy's mother, Susan, is a 7th grade school teacher in Lake City, Michigan. She is a lovely woman with a heart of gold; she cares more about her children and family than anything else in the world. She looks at all of her students as "her children." She is known in the community for volunteering to help needy children during the holidays and special needs children throughout the year.

There is only one problem: her weight. It seemed that after each child, it just took longer and longer to lose the weight. After having Jason, she bounced back pretty easily in about 3 months. After Timmy came along, it definitely took more work and about twice as much time to bounce back. Jessica was the toughest of all, it took over a year, but she still managed to do it.

Just five short years ago, she was 127 pounds, participated in many 5k runs, and was working out 3 days a week. She was confidant, assertive, and a leader in the community. On weekends she would volunteer to help special needs kids. This "giving-back" brought her great joy and a true zeal for life.

Then it happened. Don, her husband, received a phone call and due to company restructuring, or some other fancy term for cutting costs, he got laid off from his job at Specific Motors. Being laid off from the company Don thought he was going to retire with was a huge blow to him and the family. That was five years ago today.

The stress of not having as much money took a toll on everybody, but it hit Susan especially hard. She was used to getting the kids whatever they wanted, traveling once a year, and having a small vacation home on Lake Michigan.

Susan had worked hard and was happy with her lifestyle, so cutting back was not an option. She believed she could just work more, and she did. Susan quickly took on two extra part-time jobs and began working on Saturday.

The extra work helped, but it still didn't cover the amount that Don used to make at his job. To make up the difference, she ended up taking out a couple more credit cards to help pay for Christmas gifts and the vacation.

Susan just kept thinking to herself, "No big deal. He'll get his job back soon and we will get this paid off. No problem!"

Well, that never happened; he didn't get his job back. He took a couple part-time jobs before finally finding work as a long distance truck driver. He didn't make as much money, but at least it was something and he was home on the weekends to be with the family.

It was nice to have Don around on the weekends, but Susan had her hands full. With no time for herself or to volunteer anymore, she began gaining weight. At first it was barely noticeable. Susan would look in the mirror and not see any changes. Besides, most of her clothes still fit.

As the weeks progressed, Susan figured she would find a routine and things would get back to the way they used to be, but they never did.

She was constantly stressed and things just started to snowball. Her mind just kept feeding her negative thoughts. The lack of time and money were issues that led to more and more trips to fast food restaurants as well as microwave meals making their way into the fridge.

Susan didn't have time to cook, and surprisingly enough, she actually started to like the fast food that became so convenient.

Even though she couldn't really see any day-to-day changes in the mirror, her jeans didn't lie. Six months had passed and Susan could no longer fit comfortably in her clothes, so she had to replace her jeans and most of her tops.

It wasn't that big of a deal. She was no longer in her athletic running shape, but she still considered herself to be average sized compared to most of the teachers she worked with at school. This didn't bother her because when she looked around she felt fine and like she "fit in."

Unfortunately, that only lasted so long. As another year went by, those unhealthy habits that didn't seem to do much harm on a day-to-day basis started showing themselves.

Susan couldn't ignore the mirror any longer. All of those fast food and microwave meals, while easy and tasty, were catching up with her. She had gained a few more inches on her waist and she definitely did not feel like her old self.

"That's it," she told herself. "Enough is enough! I'm going to lose 10 pounds come hell or high water!" Christmas was just around the corner, so Susan decided the solution was to make a New Year's Resolution.

Don was very supportive and got her a gym membership as an early Christmas present. He knew not to mess with Susan when she put her mind to something. She had worked out regularly in the past, so Don figured it would be good for her… and he was right!

Susan began working out and started to see results. She had asked if he wanted to try to make some of the workouts with her, but Don didn't want any part of it.

After a few years of truck driving, Don had put on quite a bit of weight himself. He didn't enjoy his job, he had become overweight, and he saw no point in getting a gym membership for himself when all he was doing was driving 5-plus days a week.

Within the first week, Susan could see a difference! Not so much in the mirror, but her energy was coming back and she was elated to be getting "back on track." People took notice at school; not in how she looked, but with her endless energy levels and in how she presented herself.

Even though she wasn't back at her running weight of years past, Susan was happy to be working out again and not feeling tired all the time.

Life was good, except for one thing.

Don secretly became threatened with the new woman Susan was becoming. She had more confidence, more energy, and a newfound joy for life. He didn't like it that he wasn't experiencing any of those same feelings. The better she felt, the more they seemed to drift apart. After all, he was in a rut and misery loves company.

Just as Susan started shopping and bringing home healthier foods for the family, Don started making his own runs to the store. He wasn't on board with Susan, so he was loading up on chips, hot dogs, candy bars, and soda or whatever feel-good food he could get his hands on.

After just 4 weeks of consistently making her morning workouts, life struck again. Susan's work gave her additional responsibilities, which required her to be at work an hour earlier in the morning during what was her workout time. Unfortunately, this meant she would have to move her workouts to the evening.

Susan really believed that she would just make the evening workouts and everything would be fine, but by the time she was done teaching and working all day, she was just too tired and had to get home to feed the kids.

"I will work out tomorrow," is what she would say to herself. Sadly, it never happened.

The progress she had made during the previous month was wiped out over the next week as her energy levels and motivation plummeted. She returned to her old comfortable habits that were easy, but not very healthy in the long run. Processed food and microwave dinners replaced the healthy food and home cooked meals she had been doing.

Susan never made it past the 3-4 weeks that it typically takes to change a habit. Sadly, she didn't overcome the change at work that stole her morning workouts from her and forced her to try and workout in the evening when she had no energy. She felt like there was no solution. It was just too much to deal with. To make herself feel better, she turned to food for comfort.

Today, Susan weighs 287 pounds and has lost hope of ever being able to wear her favorite shorts again or lace up her shoes and run another 5k.

She's often thought of getting liposuction[1] but her credit cards are maxed out and she would rather have Timmy go first.

She knows Timmy gets stared at and made fun of by the other kids.

She believes that to eat healthy is too time consuming, and it doesn't taste good.

She sees skinny people and gets upset at them. She often smiles when telling her skinny friends that she was just born a "bigger girl." In reality, Susan weeps on the inside as she knows she was in great shape just a few years ago. She used to be very athletic, but those days are long gone and it would take a lot of work to get back to that point.

Susan wants to change so badly but she has failed so many times before. She has lost her confidence and her will, and now that she is so overweight, she doesn't know how to get back on track. Susan can't even exercise like she used to at this point. Taking the stairs or walking for several minutes is now a chore.

She has seen all of the miracle diets and doesn't believe for one second that any of them will work in the long term. All Susan has experienced are empty promises and "yo-yo" diets where the weight returned as quickly as it came off.

She sees shows like "The Biggest Loser" and is terrified by the yelling trainers and the pain she sees the contestants endure on a daily basis. It seems impossible, yet part of her wonders, "What if I could get my family on there? It would change our lives."

---

[1] Liposuction note: it is a common misconception that 'lipo' will help the obese. It won't. Liposuction is actually designed for people that need 'spot correction.' The maximum amount of fat you can safely remove during liposuction is 6-8 pounds. Liposuction isn't designed to go in and remove 20, 40, or even 50 pounds or more.

2

Eight Years Later

Timmy is now in college. It's his freshman year and he has never kissed a girl. He has very low self-esteem and has little, if any, social life whatsoever. Up until now, he has just assumed this is the way he was born and he blamed his parents for his being overweight.

Timmy's weight has impacted his confidence to a point where his only forms of entertainment revolve around the TV. Whether it is watching TV and movies or playing video games, Timmy doesn't leave the comfort zone that has become his living room. He would much rather have pizza delivered than venture out in public.

He hasn't decided on a major yet but feels like his purpose in life is to work on computers as an IT guy; "behind the scenes," you know.

Timmy went to a small school in Mt. Pleasant, Michigan called Central Michigan University. Aside from the fact that Timmy had forged a strong relationship with his mother who was a CMU alumni, Timmy chose CMU so he could be close to home. It was close enough where he could drive home on the weekends, but just far enough to keep his parents from dropping in on him.

You see, Timmy became the man of the house when his father was away all the time on his truck routes. He looked after his younger sister and took care of many of the family chores. Timmy really enjoyed the fulfillment that came with being a leader in the household.

When Timmy went away to college, it wasn't surprising that Jessica was depressed that her big brother was gone. She missed the talks they used to have on their way to school together. She loved talking to Timmy because it had such a calming effect on her. He could be very charismatic with people close to him.

Susan loved to go to Costco and Sam's Club and send off care packages all the time to her son at college. There was an occasion when Timmy was at class and Susan had to make a trip for work, so she snuck into his apartment and stocked it full of his favorite junk foods and sodas.

Whenever Timmy and Jason would come home for a visit, she couldn't resist stocking up her boys with all the food she had bought in bulk. Like all mothers, she loved her boys and keeping their bellies full was one thing she knew made them happy.

Unfortunately for Timmy, Mom couldn't always be there. Timmy hated college. He felt disconnected from his family and had a hard time making friends. He didn't know what it was exactly, but he lacked the confidence to speak up in class or talk to new people. He noticed people staring at him, but he didn't want to believe it was his weight. After all, his whole family was this way.

Timmy was incredibly bright and learned quickly. He was a really good listener, but very nervous to speak up if not directly called upon. Even though he was very bright, his lack of self-confidence had planted a seed in his mind that made him afraid because he assumed people were making fun of him or thinking that he was an idiot.

This insecurity held Timmy back socially and academically as he didn't believe in himself or how smart he really was.

By this time, Timmy was pushing 325 pounds and couldn't fit in most classroom desks. He tried to sit in the back corners of all his classes to minimize the amount of people that could see him. He was beginning to be self-conscious as he noticed that he wasn't like everybody else and he wasn't fitting in.

Timmy was having a lot of negative self-talk as he was walking back to his dorm. His head was down and shoulders were rolled forward; he looked sad, like a little boy whose dog ran away.

As Timmy was reaching to unlock the door to his room, his iPhone began to ring. After fumbling through his cargo pockets to chase down the elusive phone, he was finally able to get his hands on it.

He flicked his finger across the screen to answer the call…

3

Then It Happened

"Hello?" said Timmy, out of breath from walking up the flight of stairs to get to his second story apartment.

"Timmy, it's your father."

"Uh, hey Dad. How are you doing?"

Even though Timmy didn't really talk to his dad very much, he desperately wanted to have a better relationship with his father.

"Timmy, we need you to come home," Don replied flatly.

This wasn't normal behavior from his dad and it gave him an uneasy feeling in his stomach. It was the same feeling Timmy felt a few years ago when he learned that his younger sister had broken her arm on the tire swing. He just knew something was wrong.

"What is it, Dad?"

"Timmy, uh, um, it's your mother. She…uh…"

In a split second that seemed like an eternity, the knot in Timmy's stomach cinched tighter, like a boa constrictor suffocating its prey. A nervous chill shot up his spine and throughout his body, and just as Timmy's brain was starting to conjure up the worst possible scenario…

"…She had a heart attack." The rest of the words finally spilled off of his father's tongue.

Timmy was used to being the man of the house, and with that role came the necessity at times to hide or mask his emotions.

He had to be strong and set the example for his younger sister Jessica. He had to be the shoulder for her to cry on.

But this was different; this was his mother!

Timmy's arms fell to his sides, the iPhone slipping out of his hand and onto the doormat below. Tears began to shoot out of his eyes like a dam had been broken. His chubby cheeks were nothing but shiny reflective mounds coated with tears that were free flowing down his face like a waterfall.

He stood there, leaning his forehead against his door, not making any attempt to pick up the phone he had dropped. Timmy was in shock.

4

On the Road

Timmy climbed into his Chevrolet Cavalier, wondering briefly why he was still driving a car from the company that fired his dad. Timmy still blamed his dad's unhappiness and his need to be gone all the time on the fact that he got laid off from his job at Specific Motors several years ago. Don's job loss impacted the whole family.

Timmy set his backpack on the passenger seat and was just about to get situated in the driver's seat when he noticed something. Overall, the car was in ok shape, but the driver's seat looked dilapidated compared to the passenger seat. The bolsters present on the passenger seat were non-existent on the driver's side. It was completely flat and felt as if all the padding was gone.

Timmy shook his head at this most recent observation as it further reminded him that it wasn't normal to be this heavy, especially at his age. It took him a second to fasten the seatbelt as it was difficult for him to tug it across his body and then blindly try to click it in place.

Timmy turned the key and the engine sputtered to life. He had been meaning to get an oil change and a tune up but just hadn't gotten around to it. He put the car in drive and headed for home.

Timmy was not a spiritual person by any means, but like most people in times of great stress or duress, he would often turn towards God. He would pray for God to help him in times of need.

"God, please help my mom. Don't take her from me yet," he said aloud.

Oftentimes, his prayers brought him peace of mind and soothed his aching heart, but this time he didn't feel any better as he suffered much pain. The thought that his mom might not be with him anymore was almost too much for Timmy to handle.

He started to sob again like a giant 300-pound baby.

"Oh, God! Why her?! Couldn't you just TAKE ME instead? Please God...Why?" She has the biggest heart out of anyone I know!"

Just as Timmy was saying these words out loud, he had a flashback.

It was late summer and Timmy was spending time with his grandmother. His grandpa had already passed away but his Grandmother was in near-perfect physical health. She was strikingly beautiful and loved her grandchildren very much. She is the one that taught Timmy and the rest of the children in the family how to pray.

She liked to tell Timmy how to think like God thinks.

During a family vacation to the lake house several years ago, a snake bit Timmy. He and Jessica were trying to catch a frog when a snake with diamonds on its back slithered up and bit him on the leg.

Immediately, his foot swelled and he was in intense pain. Little Jessica, traumatized by the sight of her older brother in pain, ran for Grandma. When Grandma came down to where Timmy was lying, she remained completely calm. She knew 100% in her mind that Timmy was a child of God and that he could not and would not be taken by the poison. She recalled the story of Paul getting bitten in the Bible.

Grandma's calm demeanor had an immediate impact on not only Timmy, but on little Jessica who was distraught at the sight of her brother in pain. Grandma showed the children what could be accomplished in a stressful situation when you remain calm. This calmness grew out of her strong spiritual faith.

His grandma often told the kids that FEAR was merely an acronym for: False Evidence Appearing Real.

HONK! HONK!

"Hey! Watch it buddy," yelled a passing motorist.

Timmy snapped into the present at the piercing sound of the horn and the driver yelling out his window. He jerked his car to the right as he had been drifting left into oncoming traffic.

He wasn't talking on his phone or texting while driving, but his mind was clearly focused elsewhere this fateful Wednesday afternoon.

Timmy was alert again and started to think about the spiritual truths he learned from his mother and grandma.

Thoughts of the spiritual teachings he learned as a child were having a calming effect on Timmy. He began to drive a bit faster and stopped crying as he started to recite these spiritual truths.

The worry subsided but turned into a bartering act with God.

"God, if she lives, I promise I will do anything. I will be a better person. Whatever it is, you name it," said Timmy.

Timmy was willing to say, do, or trade any service with God so that he would save his mother.

"God, please hear me. I'll do anything...anything if you will heal my mom. You can't let her die!"

A notification chirp on his iPhone interrupted his thought. A text message had arrived from his dad. "Son, are you ok? It sounded like you dropped the phone. Please let me know you are ok. –Dad"

Not wanting to text while driving, Timmy plugged in his headset and called his dad to let him know he was on the road and that he would be at the hospital within an hour and a half.

Timmy sat in a trance-like state for the next 30 minutes or so. He stayed in the right hand lane with the speedometer pegged on the 65mph speed limit. As much as part of him wanted to go 100mph to get there, another part of him needed this time to think.

It wasn't until he got onto Interstate 20 about 45 minutes away from the hospital that the idea came to him that Grandma had been right all these years.

Timmy used to roll his eyes when Grandma would say, "Timmy, you are perfect just the way you are. You were made in God's eye."

Until now, Timmy had never really been a spiritual person, but this really made sense to him; at least he desperately wanted it to.

It wasn't his fault he was overweight. After all, he was God's creation; perfect, whole, and complete.

Upon recognition of his new outlook, a surge of energy shot through his veins as if he had just chugged five cans of Red Bull. For the first time in many months this surge of newfound energy brought a smile to Timmy's chubby face.

His face was round, with dimples on both cheeks and one on his chin that Grandma used to love; she would kiss her index finger then gently touch Timmy on his chin.

With this new spiritual revelation, Timmy began to think differently about his mom. She was not an obese woman that had a bad heart from all of the extra work and jobs. No, it wasn't that at all. It had nothing to do with her lifestyle and the foods she chose for herself and her family.

After all, his mom was nothing but a bundle of love, just the way God had intended her to be. God is love and so she must be made in his image and likeness. God is perfect and so is she.

This seemed so logical to Timmy that the weight he was carrying around with him started to feel more like it was meant to be a part of him instead of excess weight. He was beginning to feel lighter and better about himself; maybe there was something to this spiritual stuff that Grandma always used to talk about.

There it was off to the right hand side, a sign that read, "HOSPITAL – NEXT EXIT"

In an instant, Timmy snapped to the present. He knew that in a few minutes he would be inside the hospital learning the fate of his beloved mother.

5

A Spark of Truth

Timmy swung his Chevy Cavalier around the corner, clipping the curb with his rear tire. There, standing before him like a massive, 21st century castle was the hospital. There were no knights in shining armor here; rather doctors and nurses bustling with activity between the many buildings in their white coats and baby blue scrubs.

He slowly worked his way through the maze of concrete curbs that made up the entrance to the hospital.

Timmy had never been here and had to drive very slowly as the signs were small and there were arrows pointing all over the place. It was as if he was expecting there to be neon signs that said "Timmy's Mom" with an arrow pointing to her building.

Sadly that wasn't the case.

Having no idea where to go, he turned into a parking lot that was close to what looked like the main building.

"At least I won't have to walk far from here," Timmy thought to himself as he looked down at the badly worn soles on his shoes.

At the end of the first row was an open spot. Timmy pulled his car in headfirst, parked crooked, and with his front tires mashed up against the curb threw the gearshift lever into "park."

Before opening the door, he polished off the last Zinger and drank the remaining inch of warm Cherry Pepsi from the can that sat in the cup holder.

Timmy walked toward the hospital, craning his neck upwards to take in the enormous size of the hospital complex before entering through the massive electronic doors of the closest building.

"Bleep…bleep," chirped his iPhone.

Slightly out of breath, Timmy stopped to dig into his pocket to grab his iPhone to see who was trying to reach him. It was a text message from Jessica.

It read, "when you get here, go to the lobby of bldg C. luv u & c u soon – little j"

Timmy stopped to look around for a directory or a sign that would point him in the direction of building C. There were signs at every corner of the building he was in, but they were all medical terms pointing to different offices, labs, or rooms.

There were people walking by in all directions, but Timmy lacked the self-confidence to approach anybody and ask for help. Not to mention that his breathing was getting quite labored by this point.

"Excuse me, Sir," said a women's voice from behind him. "Are you here for the 'Lower My Health Risk' meeting today?"

Timmy scrunched his face in a look of disbelief and replied, "What are you talking about?"

The woman replied, "The 'Lower My Health Risk' is a group that meets weekly to help high risk people learn healthy living habits so they can live longer."

Timmy, still somewhat stunned and trying to catch his breath, replied, "No, I'm not here for that. I am here to see my mom. Do you know where building C is?"

The lady was polite and gave him directions to building C.

Timmy thanked her, double checked the directory at the end of the hall, and started his trek to building C.

It took Timmy about fifteen minutes to make his way to building C. He had to stop several times to catch his breath and even had to sit down for a minute at one point.

"Why does this place have to be so gosh darn big?" Timmy pondered aloud as he stood up from his short break. "I am only doing this walk for you Mom," Timmy muttered under his breath as he continued on.

Even though Timmy was out of breath and hated the fact that he had to walk so far on his trek through the hospital complex, he was like a sponge, soaking up his new surroundings. He was trying to take in and process all of the activity going on around him.

There were two things that stood out to Timmy on his walk. It wasn't the technology or the modern design of the hospital; it was a realization that hit him like a ton of bricks. Most of the people that he saw as patients in the hospital were either elderly or overweight.

In a sense, this made him comfortable because he saw a lot of people like him, but at the same time there was a slight uneasiness that came over him. Was this merely a simple observation, or was there a hint of truth to the matter that overweight people had more health problems?

"Am I on the same path as these people?" Timmy thought to himself.

Timmy pondered it for a second before he was interrupted by a familiar voice.

"You made it!" exclaimed Jessica, who managed to wipe away her tears just long enough to welcome her favorite big brother.

Don was just down the hall, pacing back and forth with his head down. He did manage to look up just long enough to make eye contact with Timmy and acknowledge his presence, then he disappeared around the corner.

Jessica locked onto Timmy with a big hug as she was looking to him for strength. Timmy was holding her head with his hand, gently brushing her hair while telling her everything was going to be OK.

As they were holding their embrace, Don came back around the corner. He had just bought some snacks for the two of them: Doritos for Jessica and Timmy's all-time favorite, Ho-Ho's.

Looking up from his embrace with Jessica, Timmy quickly replied, "No thanks, Dad. I'm full."

Don looked surprised; it was normal for Timmy to eat one or two packages in one sitting. Timmy was even known to eat them for breakfast sometimes!

Don shrugged, opened the package, and ate both Ho-Ho's in four quick bites. He was hungry as he hadn't eaten since taking Susan to the Hospital, and he didn't know when he was going to eat next.

Just then, a tall lanky figure approached. He wore blue scrubs and a white coat like everybody else, but there was something special about this guy. You just wanted to stop what you were doing and look at him. It's hard to explain, but the man commanded respect.

Extending his right hand, he said, "Mr. Johnston, I am Doctor Hammond. I have been taking care of Mrs. Johnston."

Timmy and Jessica ended their embrace, quickly wiped the drying tears from their eyes, and turned their attention towards Don and Dr. Hammond.

Dr. Hammond acknowledged Timmy and Jessica and said, "Your mother is going to be ok. She is a very strong person, but she is also very lucky. Most people I see in her shape would have passed away already. That is why she is going into surgery right away."

Then he said something that stuck with Timmy, "It's like someone was watching out for her."

Those were the Doctor's exact words.

Timmy became insanely grateful. Intent on honoring the deal he made to God while driving to the hospital, Timmy was going to lose weight and help his family do the same thing. After all, he is the one that made the barter less than three hours ago; he couldn't break it now just because his mom was going to be ok.

Timmy knew that he was destined for greatness, and if he were going to help this world he would have to lose weight and be in better physical shape. He committed to himself that he was going to make a change and see it through!

After all, his family depended on it!

6

On a Mission

Jason had made it to the hospital later that Wednesday evening after Susan was out of surgery. The family stayed together to support one another until they brought Mom home Sunday morning.

Susan's surgery went well, and she stayed in the hospital for those extra days to make sure there were no complications and that she was stable and ready to go home.

Timmy wanted to take the week off of school to be there to care for his mother, but she wouldn't have any of it.

"Timmy, I'm fine! What I need is for you to be in school getting an education so that you can go on in life to do great things."

"But Mom, you almost died! I want to help you get healthy so we never have to go through this again. Plus, I promised God that I would lose weight and help you lose weight too if you lived," exclaimed Timmy.

"Come here, Timmy, and give me a big hug. You know I would never leave you or this family."

"I know Mom, but we were all very scared for you."

"I understand that Timmy, and I'm sorry. But since you made a promise to God and to yourself, I think you need to get your behind back to college tomorrow so you can start fulfilling the promises that you made."

"You're right Mom. I am going to go to school and see what help and resources are available to me. Then I can share my knowledge with you guys so we don't have to go through this again. Mom, it was really scary seeing all the overweight people in the hospital. I know we don't have the 'skinny gene,' but we need to do something about our health."

"You are right. This was definitely an eye-opening experience for me, too. The thought of dying and leaving the four of you behind has really been weighing on my mind. Dr. Hammond and the nurse gave me a basic list of things I need to be doing, but I want you to find out all you can about healthy lifestyles. I was very scared lying on that table in the operating room, and I don't want anybody to have to go through that," replied Susan.

A big smile came across Timmy's face as he had a powerful feeling again; he was going to be not just the man of the house, but also the man that was going to save the house.

Timmy spent a few minutes packing for his return trip to school so he could spend the rest of the afternoon with his family. It was good to have Jessica, Jason, and his dad there with him.

Timmy thought to himself, "It sucks that it took Mom almost dying to get the family close together again. I know we are all busy, but we should never be too busy for each other."

With that thought, Timmy knew that his losing weight would be cause for the rest of the family to join in. Not only would it make everybody healthier, but it would also get the family close together and strengthen their bond.

Timmy stayed through dinner before heading back to school that evening. Not only did he want to spend more time with his family, but he also wanted to make sure that his mom ate a healthy dinner like the doctor ordered.

At about 8pm, Timmy said his goodbyes and began his drive back to school. Normally he would be dreading a Monday, and all of the classes that go with it, but this time was different. Timmy had a promise to keep and he was excited to see what resources the college had available to help him.

He knew he had a lot of work in store for him, but after facing the prospect of losing his mom, he knew there wasn't an alternative. As much as Timmy feared the loss of his mother, deep down inside he knew that he could be following in her footsteps if he didn't change his ways.

He kept thinking back to the lady who asked if he was part of the "Lower My Health Risk" group that was meeting at the hospital. He knew that she was only trying to help, but it bothered him to no end that he fit the profile as a "high health risk" person.

Timmy was going to change and that is all there was to it. All he needed was the right people and information to help him. He was excited for Monday morning because he was going to go see one of the school counselors about the resources available to help him.

Timmy made it back to school safely. No honking horns or drifting lanes this time around. The only drifting occurred when he got home and his head hit the pillow, and he drifted off to sleep.

7

In Search of Change

BUZZ... BUZZ... BUZZ.

It was 6:30am and Timmy's alarm was going off. Instead of snoozing the requisite 3-5 times like he usually did each day, he rolled out of bed, ready to start the day and be the first person in line at the counselor's office.

Instead of polishing off a package of Zingers for breakfast, Timmy took the time to go to the cafeteria where he ate a bowl of cereal with low-fat milk instead.

Normally, he avoided the cafeteria because people just stared at him. Today he didn't care. This was the first day of the new Timmy, and he knew it was only going to be a matter of time until he was back to a normal weight.

It was 7:30am and Timmy was standing outside of the counselor's office waiting for them to arrive. Not thirty seconds later, the door opened and a very charismatic red headed Irish man stepped out.

"Hi, my name is John. How may I help you today? If you need schedule changes or career assistance, you will need to come back later as I am not the one that handles those things," said the friendly man to Timmy.

"No, no, I don't need any of those things. Actually, what I need is to talk to somebody or see what resources are available for me to learn about healthy living and losing weight," replied Timmy.

"What is your name?"

"Oh sorry, my name is Timmy." He extended his right hand to shake John's hand.

John slowly looked up and down Timmy, nodded his head, and asked him to come into his office. You see, John had once suffered from being obese as well, and he could see the determination in his eyes and hear the desperation in his voice. Timmy was determined to make a change, but also desperate for the guidance to do so.

John asked, "Timmy, what exactly is going on? I can see in your eyes a sense of urgency. Why is this so important to you now?"

Timmy looked John in the eyes and began to tell the story of the past week and how he thought he was going to lose his mother to a heart attack.

He told John how he would have given up his own life for her. He even went back to his childhood and talked about his upbringing. He told John of the amazing woman that brought him into this world and how she always wanted the best for him.

She would never do anything to intentionally hurt him or the rest of the family, but Timmy finally realized that over the years, his mom got busy and lost sight of the importance of eating healthy food. She was misled by millions of dollars of marketing and had assumed all of the convenient and "fast" food was healthy.

John thanked Timmy for his honesty and openness, but also wanted to remind him that it was all in the past. The only thing they could do now was work on the present and look toward the future. John reminded Timmy that the important thing was that Susan was making a strong recovery.

Timmy nodded in agreement.

John took a deep breath before confiding in Timmy that at one point in his life he battled obesity.

Timmy's eyes lit up as he found somebody that he could actually relate to. When looking at John, obesity is the last thing that came to Timmy's mind. This gave him great confidence inside, and a smile began to cross his lips.

Timmy told John of the deal he had made with God. He told John that it was up to him to not only change himself, but also his family and others. Then it hit him like a ton of bricks, "Maybe my purpose is much bigger than just me and my family. Maybe my purpose is to help all the people battling weight issues and obesity," he thought to himself.

John smiled as it brought back memories of when he decided to make the same life changes himself.

"Timmy, I see great things for you, and I will do whatever I can to help. When I look at you, I see my old self from many years ago."

"Before we really get moving, I want to talk to you about putting a plan in place. There is more than just 'losing weight' that we have to deal with. We want to look at all aspects of your life and make everything better, not just your body. Are you committed to changing your life for the better?"

"Wow, that sounds amazing," said Timmy. "I am totally committed, and I can't believe how lucky I am!"

"Timmy, I want to meet with you in person about once a week, and I want you to feel free to email or call me as well," said John.

"One last thing, since you are apart from your family and can only see them on occasional weekends, I want you to write letters to your mom letting her know what you are learning.

"This serves several purposes. One: I always found that I learned a subject better when I had to teach somebody else what I had learned. Two: if you are sending letters to your mother, there is no way she is going to let you down. It will help her and the rest of your family stay on track. Finally, writing those letters to your mom will make you feel great and it will remind you of your bigger purpose.

"How does that sound?"

"Excellent," responded Timmy enthusiastically.

"Great, now I want you to write a letter to your mom letting her know what she is going to have to look forward to. You know, Timmy, mothers always love to get letters from their boys!"

"Sounds good John, I will get on it!"

"I want you to come back on Wednesday, as there is somebody special that I want you to meet. This person will be helping you with losing weight and adopting a healthy lifestyle. I will be helping you with the other aspects of your life. Get that letter out to your mom, and I will see you Wednesday!"

"Thank you sooooo much John!"

Timmy left John's office, hopped on the shuttle, and went back to his dorm to write his letter to Mom before his first class later in the morning.

8

Letter to Mom #1

Monday, September 6

Dear Mom,
    I hope you are doing well. Even though I just left the house yesterday, I really miss you. I'm grateful Dad took some time off to be with you during your recovery. I'm grateful you are alive.

    You know I wasn't too excited to go back to school because I wanted to spend the week taking care of you. Well, as luck (or God) would have it, I met an amazing counselor today.

    His name is John; he is a funny Irish man with an authentic Irish accent. His mannerisms remind me of Uncle David. What's cool is that he understands what it is like to be heavy. There was a time in his life when he was severely overweight, but looking at him now you would never know.

    He is going to help me in all aspects of my life, not just in losing weight. I get to meet with him every week so that I stay on track. He has a 'surprise' person for me to meet on Wednesday as well. I have no idea what he has in store for me, but I am looking forward to it!

    One of the things he wants me to do is to write to you often. This will not only help our communication, but it will be very educational for you and the rest of the family. John says it will help me learn better if I have to teach you what I am learning. He said the material will be beneficial to you living a healthier life. After all, it isn't just about me losing weight. Our family needs to be healthy so we are there for one another for many years to come.

So, be prepared to get lots of letters from me, Mom. I'm going to be busy improving myself and sharing my knowledge with you. Please do what the doctor says and continue on a healthy path! I want you to be around when I have grandkids one day.

Love,

Your son, Timmy

9

Timmy and the Trainer

Timmy sat up in his bed. It was still 15 minutes before his alarm was supposed to go off, but Timmy was excited about this Wednesday and what John would have in store for him.

Since their meeting on Monday, Timmy had spent quite a bit of time online researching information on eating right, working out, and living a healthy lifestyle.

In a sense, he was excited about what he was seeing, but at the same time he was experiencing some information overload.

There was just so much information on Google that the more he read, the less he thought he knew and the more confused he became. He was having a hard time separating the good information from all of the marketing hype, quick fixes, and miracle pills that seemed to be available.

Through his many searches, Timmy was able to find a group that he learned from and enjoyed. It was a Facebook group that posted lots of short videos and information about living a healthy lifestyle. He joined the "Fit Life (Think, Feel, and Become)" Group because they kept things simple and fostered an environment that was supportive with members that were open to sharing and helping others.

Timmy even overcame his shyness enough to post a comment on their page about his situation and how much their short videos were helping him.

Realizing he only had about 45 minutes until his meeting with John, Timmy decided to head to the cafeteria to get some breakfast.

At first it was tough for Timmy to not eat all of the junk and snack cakes that had been around him. Now he would just settle for a big bowl of cereal with low-fat milk. He knew it wasn't a complete breakfast, but it was a big improvement over what he had been doing.

After only drinking whole milk his entire life, he was initially worried about trying the low-fat milk, but he really couldn't tell much difference when it was on his cereal. He just assumed it was healthier because it was called low-fat.

Timmy finished his cereal quickly because unlike past times where he would just take the campus shuttle to get around, today he was going to walk, even though he usually got out of breath and long walks hurt his feet. He guessed it was probably a quarter-mile away or so and gave himself about 15-20 minutes to get there.

This was a big step for Timmy. When you weigh over 300 pounds, it hurts to walk for more than a minute or two. His ankles would be sore, along with his knees and lower back.

While walking to John's office, Timmy's mind was racing, wondering what special surprise John had in store for him. With his mind a flurry of activity, he didn't feel any pain during the walk and even managed to walk there in under 15 minutes.

Timmy walked into the office and this time he was greeted by John's administrative assistant, Sandy.

"Hi Timmy," she chirped in a perky voice that had a tiny hint of a sweet Southern accent. "I'm Sandy, John's assistant. He is really looking forward to your meeting this morning. Please, follow me."

"Uh...uh...ok," stammered Timmy.

He thought he was out of breath from the walk over, but after seeing Sandy and hearing her voice, he realized that she took his remaining breath away.

Timmy knew she could tell how nervous he was, but there was nothing he could do about it. He really hadn't had much interaction with people outside of his family and his teachers at school. Timmy realized he needed to work on being comfortable around people if he was ever going to enjoy social situations.

Sandy led Timmy to John's office.

As soon as the door opened up, John popped his head up.

"What's going on, buddy?" said an energetic John in his thick Irish accent.

Timmy couldn't help but smile. Something about John's voice and confident nature just lit him up. He wanted to be confident like that someday as well.

"I'm well. I just walked over from the cafeteria. Longest walk I have taken in a while."

"That is great to hear! Timmy, I want you to meet a great friend of mine, Matthew."

As far as Timmy could tell, Matthew was in near perfect physical shape and looked like a gladiator or an action figure of sorts. He was wearing jeans and a V-neck t-shirt, but you could tell he had strong arms, shoulders, chest and whatever those muscles are that bulge up when you shrug your shoulders* (*trapezius muscle, "traps" for short, he would soon learn).

Timmy couldn't get over how the t-shirt just hung on his body. Matthew looked like a statue, and Timmy was impressed. This guy obviously knew a thing or two about staying in shape.

"Hello, Timmy," said Matthew confidently.

Timmy was still somewhat blown away by the surprise that John had for him, so he only managed to stutter, "N...N..Nice to m...m..meet you too."

"John told me a little bit about your situation, and thought we should meet. I would be more than happy to set aside a block of time every week for us to get together. That is, if you are up for it?"

A huge smile crossed Timmy's face. He was excited like a little kid on Christmas morning. "Up for it, are you kidding me? I will do whatever you need me to do. After all, my life, and the lives of my family members depend on it."

"That's great," said Matthew, with a smile crossing his face. "I have spent some time talking to John, and here is what we would like to do. You will meet with John on Mondays, and you will meet with me on Wednesdays. John is going to work with you on personal and life challenges, and I am going to work with you on your health and nutritional challenges."

Timmy nodded.

"Together we are going to show you how to become the confident, healthy, outgoing person that is hidden away inside you.

That's right, Timmy, it is inside you right now; we just have to uncover it and pull it out of you."

"Matthew is right. We are going to make it as easy and straightforward as possible for you, but it will take some effort and commitment on your part," said John.

"We are here for you 100%, Timmy, and we want you to be healthy and live a long and fulfilling life. That said, are you prepared to commit to do the things we tell you to do?" asked Matthew.

"Yes! I will do whatever it takes. Almost losing my mom was a huge eye opener for me. Not only that, but when I look in the mirror, I see myself going down that same road, and it really scares me. I know I need to change," replied Timmy.

"Sounds good," said Matthew.

"I know you have a lot of free time today, so that is why I scheduled Wednesdays to be your day to spend time with Matthew," said John.

"I have another meeting to attend to, so I am going to leave the two of you alone to get started. Thanks, guys."

"Timmy, here is how I want to go about things. John has told me a lot about your situation, so the first thing I want to do is talk to you about the obesity problem in general. I have found it tough to tackle solutions without first discussing the problem, how it came to be, and the effects.

"Once we break things down and have a good understanding of the issue at hand, we will then work together to overcome each issue one by one.

"I have found it is a lot easier to break big problems down into smaller, more manageable pieces, and then work to correct things one by one. I like to take the overwhelming, like trying to lose 100 pounds, and turn it into something manageable like losing one pound per week. Which one seems easier to you, Timmy?"

"Well, obviously, losing one pound per week seems much more attainable than trying to lose 100 pounds."

"Exactly! After all, it isn't just your health that is going to be impacted. You are going to help your family as well, which I know is very important to you."

"Want to know something else Timmy?"

"Sure, what's that?"

"You are going to become an ambassador. You are going to be able to take what you have learned and use it to help and teach others as I am doing with you. This is going to be way bigger than just you and your family."

A smile crossed Timmy's face as he sat up straighter in his seat. The "new" Timmy was already starting to uncover himself.

10

Getting Bigger...Little by Little

"Before we get going here, I want you to know that you can stop me at any point if you have questions or need me to clarify things. Sound good?"

Timmy nodded his head in approval as he got out a pen and notebook.

"Great! Let's get moving," said Matthew. "How many people do you know now or in the past that have had issues with gaining weight, but didn't really know how it happened?"

Timmy shrugged.

"At least a few I am sure."

Timmy nodded in agreement.

"Maybe it was a friend or relative you only saw a few times a year. You probably noticed they had put on a few pounds since the last time you saw them, but that was only because you only saw them every 6 to 8 months.

"It is tougher to spot weight gain when you are around the person on a regular basis. Most people don't know or realize they are gaining weight until it is something drastic like trying on an old pair of pants or a dress they haven't worn in months or years."

Timmy looked at Matthew, taking in every word, his head bobbing in agreement with most of what was being said.

"Nobody puts on 30 pounds in a month. It is a slow 1-2 pounds per month that, over the course of a year or several years, quietly turns into that spare tire or extra weight that I help people to lose."

"Hey Matthew, do you mind if I interrupt for a second?"

"No, not at all, Timmy. What is it?"

"When I was about ten or eleven years old, I was over 200 pounds. Here we are nine or ten years later and I am close to 325 pounds. That means I was only putting on 12-15 pounds each year, which doesn't sound as bad when you break that down to a pound or so a month that I was gaining."

"You're exactly right, Timmy. You were getting bigger, little by little. But it wasn't just you; it was our entire country."

Matthew pulled out a sheet of paper.

"In case you haven't seen the latest statistics, here they are: out of the top 33 developed nations on the globe, America is now the most overweight country in the developed world. About 34% of the US population over age 20 is obese, 33% is overweight, and another 5% is extremely or morbidly obese," read Matthew from the article.

"The really scary thing is what is happening to our children. Childhood obesity has more than tripled in the past 30 years. The prevalence of obesity among children aged 6 to 11 years increased from 6.5% in 1980 to 19.6% in 2008. The prevalence of obesity among adolescents aged 12 to 19 years increased from 5.0% to 18.1%. (http://www.cdc.gov/HealthyYouth/obesity/)

"I found my purpose in life, and it is helping people like yourself make lifestyle changes so that you can be free to enjoy all that life has to offer. You don't have to be hostage to your weight any longer."

Timmy thought to himself about all the things he hadn't been able to do because of his weight. He never went on water skiing or wakeboarding trips over the summer, or ski trips during the winter. He avoided going to the beach or hanging out by the swimming pool in the summer.

Matthew's voice finally made him snap out of his brief trance.

"There are some simple reasons why we are this predicament as a country.

"First off, I don't believe that 70% of our country is just lazy. I know that is what some mean people like to say about overweight people, but I don't believe that one bit. I believe that work, family, technology, and a gradual development and acceptance of poor nutrition habits got us where we are today.

"Like you just realized on your own, Timmy, you were only putting on a pound or so each month, but do that for two, five, or even ten years or more, and it is easy to see how our obesity rate got so high.

"That said, I want to help everybody that doesn't want to live this way any longer. I want to help people make subtle lifestyle changes that will give them a more rewarding and fulfilling life.

"I hear it all the time. 'I was in great shape in high school; I put on a few pounds in college, but nothing big. I have always been normal or in shape. Then I got busy with work and the family…' and you know the rest of the story. In fact, I'm pretty sure this story might hit close to home for you, Timmy."

Timmy looked at Matthew, nodding slowly.

"What about your mom and dad? John told me that your family has always been 'heavier,' but it sounds like there was a time when your mom used to be pretty athletic and your dad was in pretty good shape."

"Yes, that is true."

"Then life happened with regards to jobs and work, which ended up changing those habits. I know that your dad had to become a truck driver and, besides the fact that he didn't like the job, sitting all day is hard. I know that your mom had to take on several jobs to help replace your dad's lost income."

"You are right, Matthew. I thought we were always heavy, but looking back, there was a time when Mom was in great shape. When dad lost his job, I think that is when our habits really changed. My parents became busy, always tired, and not happy like they used to be. I believe that is when things really changed for our family."

"Do you think you have what it takes to turn back the clock for your family? They are going to look to you for leadership and guidance."

"I don't know."

"Well, you do have what it takes. Don't worry, I am going to coach you through the whole thing."

"That sounds great!" replied Timmy with excitement.

"Instead of putting on that silent and sneaky 1-2 pounds per month, I am going to teach you how to strip off anywhere from one to six pounds per month WITHOUT any drastic changes to your life.

"But what if I want to lose more weight faster?" asked Timmy.

"That is a great question, and one that I love to hear.

"You see, Timmy, I want to help people get back to a healthy weight. I don't expect people who have never worked out or eaten properly in a long time to all of a sudden make big, drastic changes. I can't expect somebody that hasn't worked out in years to become some crazy workout or fitness person. It happens, but it just isn't realistic, and it isn't going to resonate with many people."

"Ok, so then what is your goal?"

"My goal is to help everybody lose weight by giving them tools and letting them decide how much or how little they want to do. The important thing is that no matter what, they will get there eventually. If I can get enough people to make a few small changes to their lives so instead of gaining a pound per month, they are losing a pound a month, that is a big victory."

"That makes sense. It is just different than what most programs say. It seems most diets give you some super strict program that has to be strictly followed or it won't work. At least that is what I saw with my mom when she tried a few diets."

"Exactly, but I will tell you this, it always makes my day when somebody like you comes along and basically says, 'Crawling is nice, but I want to walk and run.' Losing the weight slowly with minimal life changes is nice, but hearing that somebody is motivated to make real life changes makes my job worth it.

"I understand that you are busy. I know your blackberry and iPhone don't stop vibrating, flashing, and going off all day. I know you have school, work, chores, and a million other distractions throughout your day.

"Trust me, I GET it!"

Timmy smiled as he could see and hear the passion in Matthew's voice and body language.

"I know you have better things to do than workout all day, and with the demands of life, work, and family, nobody blames you! It isn't your fault."

"Really?"

"No, it really isn't, Timmy. You got your habits from your parents when you were very young. It was all you knew. As you got older, you were influenced by government-sanctioned food pyramids at school and by commercials and advertising everywhere else you went. None of these things are going to teach you good, life-long, healthy habits.

"It takes healthy parents or a role model; it takes somebody showing and helping you to develop good eating habits so that you can live a healthy life. I was fortunate to grow up with two parents that lived a healthy lifestyle.

"Now you are getting me as your role model. But don't worry; it isn't too late. You are still very young and have a long, fulfilling life ahead of you.

"How does that make you feel?"

"Honestly, I feel much better. I keep looking at myself as needeing to lose 100+ pounds, and it seemed like an insurmountable task; but after talking to you and seeing that I got that way by putting on one lowly pound per month, it seems attainable to reach a normal weight."

"I like your attitude!" exclaimed Matthew. "Let's take a break and get a glass of water, and we will keep going if you would like."

"Yes, I would love to keep going. I am really learning a lot already."

Matthew and Timmy left the office and headed down the hall towards the restrooms and water fountain.

11

America's Biggest Crisis – A Lack of Movement

"Nothing better than taking a break, getting a nice stretch in, and having a glass of water; what do you think, Timmy?"
"You know, Matthew, the water was actually pretty refreshing. I normally don't drink just plain water. I have a question though, I didn't see you do any stretching, did I miss something?"

"Water is so healthy and refreshing to the body, I now drink it more than anything else. As far as the stretching goes, I developed a stretch to stop lower back pain that you can do anywhere, and the cool thing is that nobody can tell you are doing it! I call it 'The Squeeze.' Don't worry, we will cover this in a little bit."

"Very cool, I can't wait!"
"Are you ready to keep learning?"
"You bet I am!" replied Timmy.
"Great. Let's get started.

"Before we can begin to correct something, it helps to know the problem or issue that needs correcting. In America's case, a major issue is a lack of movement.

"We live in a country that has always prided itself on being bigger and better, but it is time we shift those priorities and realize that not everything is better by being bigger. Deficits and waistlines are two things that we could definitely stand to shrink a bit."

Timmy chuckled out loud.

"We now live in a country where over 70 percent of the adult population is overweight or obese.

"Our expanding waistlines are to the point now where the government and the media call it an 'obesity epidemic' because the problem is increasing so fast and affecting so many people."

Timmy looked at Matthew sheepishly.

"Timmy, this problem didn't happen overnight; it is one of those problems that has crept up on us. Just like an individual that slowly puts on 15 pounds a year, they have no real idea until they try on that old pair of jeans that used to fit so well, or they see pictures from the past and realize they don't look the same anymore.

"I bet you saw the same thing with your parents. John said there was a period of time when your mom got busy at work because a big project came up, or something like that. When it happened, she wasn't able to work out at the gym anymore, she ate out a few more times than normal, and she even started to bring the fast food home on the way from work."

"Yes, that happened."

"I am sure your mom thought, 'no big deal, I don't see any difference,' at least in the short term."

"You're good, Matthew. I never really looked at it that way as it was several years ago and I was much younger. But I do remember my mom starting to work out for a few weeks there. I remember it because there was a noticeable shift in her energy levels. She was upbeat, happy, and had a positive energy about her."

"What happened next?" probed Matthew.

"I don't remember the specifics, but Mom got overloaded at work and couldn't make her morning workouts. But what I do remember, because I really liked it, was the fact that she would bring home McDonald's, pizza, or other takeout food several nights a week. Boy was it tasty!"

"I see. Did your mom ever go back to working out?"

"No. Work changes meant no more morning workouts, and she never got into a routine with the evening workouts."

"Sadly, that is how it starts for so many people. Like your mom, they never get back on schedule. Most people mean to get back on track, but as one project ends, another begins.

"I hear it all the time; 'I know I need to exercise and eat better, but I got busy with work/family/school. I can't see a difference, so I will just keep going.'

"You know what happens because you lived it. Pretty soon the old habits have been replaced by new habits, which in most cases are not as healthy. These new habits don't have an immediate visible impact; it takes a while to notice.

"Then one day, months down the road, you are standing in the mirror going 'I don't remember these pants (or dress) being so tight.' Probably not, because like I will show you, little things over time can make a big difference. The real problem is that over those months, you ingrained a new set of unhealthy habits into your mind and body that will have to be overcome."

"Hold on a second, Matthew."

"Ok, what is it, Timmy?"

"Well, we had bad habits as a family for many years. Does that mean it is going to take us years to turn things around?"

"Don't worry, Timmy; it isn't going to take years to turn things around. It might take some time to lose all the weight you want to lose, but as far as the habits go, you will need about a month to replace your old habits with new ones. Don't worry; with the help of a program I like to call *The Lean Life*, I am going to help you turn it all around!"

"Whew! I was worried it was going to take five or ten years to change those habits."

"Not at all, Timmy. Let's move forward and take a look at the typical American day.

"When I am going through this example, Timmy, I want you think if this sounds like what your mom and dad were doing on a daily basis. I know this example is pretty simplistic, but I am using it to illustrate a point. Here is an example of the 'typical American day.' We will use the fictional character Jane for this example, but it could be anybody."

Matthew pulled out a handout with writing and pictures on it, and sat down next to Timmy.

"Let's take a look at this together."

- *Jane wakes up.*

- She walks to the kitchen where she sits down for a few minutes to eat breakfast. Back rounded, shoulders hunched over, chin and neck pushing forward. Like this:

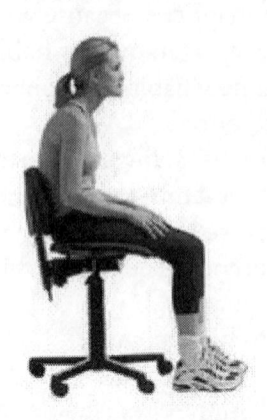

Then she walks to the garage to sit in the car so she can drive to work for 20-90 minutes.

"Wait a second," said Timmy. "People actually commute to work for an hour or more?"

"Believe it or not, yes. Sixty to ninety minute commutes are the norm for many people in California and other congested metropolitan areas like DC, Atlanta, Chicago, New York, etc."

- Notice the rounded back, shoulders hunched over, chin and neck pushing forward. Like this:

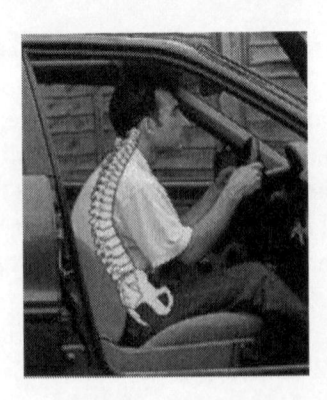

Once Jane arrives at work, she will probably drive around for three to five minutes to find the closest parking spot to save herself from having to walk *very far. She does the same thing at the mall or when running errands to the grocery or shopping center.*

Timmy's eyes dart away from Matthew and he tries to conceal a smile.

"I know it happens, because I see it all the time. I am the guy that grabs an open spot and starts walking so I can get on with my day and get in a little bit of exercise.

"I see the smile on your face Timmy; you know exactly what I am talking about. How many times have you seen somebody sit there with their blinker on, waiting for somebody to load their car from the grocery, when there are open spots literally three to five parking spaces away?

"I used to find it funny, but now that we are having an obesity epidemic due partly to a 'movement crisis' in our country, I find it sad. I am here to help people see the value in changing those habits."

Timmy nodded in agreement.

"Back to our typical day."

- Once at work, Jane will park her caboose in a nice office chair and stare at a computer screen for the better part of the day. Again, back rounded, shoulders hunched over, chin and neck pushing forward. Like this:

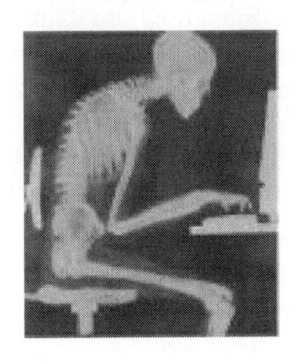

Jane will walk to the water cooler or rest room, or out to take a smoke break, but for the most part, she will be sitting down for many hours during the day.

- Time for lunch. Jane will probably head to a) the local fast food joint, b) the local 'quick food' restaurant (TGI Fridays, Applebee's, etc.), or c) enjoy a nice 'Lean Cuisine' or other microwave meal. Jane likes the microwave meals because eating out gets expensive, and the microwave meals don't take long to prepare.

- Jane should be happy because it is 5pm and time to go home, but she is too exhausted and tired. Exhausted from a day where she sat on her behind for 8 hours and didn't walk more than a hundred yards.

- It's a good thing Jane got that great parking spot; she didn't have to walk very far to the car. Again, she sits for another 20-90 minutes in rush-hour traffic on the way home. (Back rounded, shoulders hunched over, chin and neck pushing forward. I don't think I need to insert another pic.)

- Yay! Jane made it home in record time, but she is too tired to celebrate the small victory. She is still thinking about the two red lights she got stuck at, but missed the fact she made the other ten green ones.

"Don't worry, Timmy; we will work on creating a positive mindset in a future lesson. You can't learn everything at once."

- Jane gets out of the car and heads into the kitchen where it is time for dinner. Since the day was so exhausting, she doesn't feel like cooking anything, so she resorts to the same 'convenient' options: microwave dinners, frozen pizza, and other pre-packaged food that can be prepared in the oven.

- Upon sitting down at the dinner table (Again, back rounded, shoulders hunched over, chin and neck pushing forward. ARE WE STARTING TO SEE A PATTERN HERE?), Jane shares how exhausted she is and how tiring her day was. When the meal is complete and the dishes are put away, Jane heads to the couch where she can relax in front of the TV for a few hours.

"Do you want to guess how she is sitting?"

"Sure," says Timmy, rolling his eyes. "Back rounded, shoulders hunched over, with her chin and neck pushing forward."

"Exactly. See how quickly you learn with a little repetition? The same thing applies to habits with your body."

- Jane finishes watching another exciting episode of the Biggest Loser. 'At least I am not like those people,' she thinks to herself. Time for bed as Jane has another busy day tomorrow.

- Jane gets up from her comfortable couch and walks to the bedroom where she lies down, hoping to get a good night's sleep.

"So Timmy, how did I do for a simplistic example of the typical American day? I saw you smile a few times, so I am sure there were a few things you could relate to."

"Sounds pretty typical to me, Matthew. There were definitely a few things that made me smile. I am sure that many people would be able to relate to Jane."

"Yes, it was overly simplistic, but at the same time I saw you nodding your head in agreement on several occasions. I am guessing that most people will see aspects of Jane's day in their own lives, or in the lives of their friends and family.

"Remember how I kept saying and exaggerating 'back rounded, shoulders hunched over, chin and neck pushing forward,' into the story?"

"Let me guess, you have a reason for that?"

"Of course I do," said Matthew with a grin.

"Even if you don't believe the statistics that most people spend about 90% of their day sitting or lying down, I am going to show you the cumulative effects of having the poor body positioning mentioned above. I am going to explain to you how to spot the effects of those postures and what you can do to correct them."

"Ok, but what does this have to do with being overweight?"

"Great question. Let me ask you something."

"Ok."

"I noticed the uneven wear on the soles of your shoes, and I want to know if it is comfortable walking in those shoes?"

"You noticed the bottom of my shoes? What does that have to do with anything?"

"I am glad you asked. The highly slanted angle and the uneven wear on the soles of your shoes is caused largely by your posture, Timmy."

"Really?" said Timmy with a puzzled look on his face as he stared down at his shoes.

"Yes. We have a crisis in movement in this country and it is not only impacting waistlines, but it is impacting our posture as well. This poor posture impacts the ability to live pain-free, which in turn makes movement harder.

"It kind of becomes a catch-22 as having poor posture makes it hard to move and do even the basic types of exercise necessary to lose weight."

A serious look crossed Timmy's face.

"I have to be honest with you; I noticed the wear on my shoes the other day as it hurts my feet to walk. The soles are worn at such an angle; I don't know what to do. Even when I get new shoes, it doesn't take long for them to end up like this.

"That said, do you think we can take another break and get some water before we keep going?"

"You read my mind. During our break let's take a short walk and get some water before we look at the posture issues caused by a lack of movement. How does that sound?"

"Perfect," replied Timmy.

12

Stop Lower Back Pain and Start Losing Weight

"Hey Matthew, I think I saw you stretching again on the break. When are you going to teach me how to do it?"

A smile crossed Matthew's chiseled face.

"It makes me so happy to work with somebody that is excited to learn and change their life. Just have a little more patience as we are almost there."

"Ok," sighed Timmy. "I just really want to learn how to lose this weight."

"I completely understand your desire to lose weight, but before you can focus on losing weight, there are some underlying fundamentals you need to understand.

"I could take the easy road and just give you a series of workouts to do and turn you loose, just hoping you would succeed. I don't take shortcuts with people, though, as that would be the wrong thing to do. Not to mention you would most likely injure yourself, which would set you back even further."

Timmy sat there in silence, digesting the fact that Matthew really cared about his well-being, and that he had a plan.

"We both know it took you ten plus years to get where you are today. I think we both agree we can't change that overnight, but I am telling you we can change things quickly.

"I know we all want instant gratification, but that isn't a reality. The reality is, if you put action into the things you are about to learn, then you will reach your goals. More importantly, I am going to show you how to do it safely and without injury. The last thing I want is for you to get injured and then get discouraged."

"I know, I know," replied Timmy with a sheepish look on his face. He knew Matthew had a plan, but his eagerness and impatience was getting the better of him. "I apologize. I know I need to be patient."

"It's ok, Timmy; patience isn't my strong suit either. We are almost there, but first I need to teach you about several important postural deficiencies that stem from the 'crisis in movement' that we just discussed.

"The first issue I want to cover affects about eighty percent of the adult population at one time or another. I am sure you have heard your parents or other people you know complain of lower back pain."

"Yes, most definitely," replied a perked up Timmy.

"Since lower back pain affects so many people and is one that I feel most people can relate to, I will use lower back pain to demonstrate how the body works, and then I will show you how to prevent or minimize lower back pain. As you can imagine, it is hard to walk or do any type of exercise if your back hurts.

"The good news is that on your way to stopping your lower back pain, you will end up correcting several other key posture issues as well. This is sort of like killing five birds with one stone!"

"What are the other posture issues?"

"We will get to those in just a bit. But as a hint, think back to what we discussed with the crisis in movement. That should give you a pretty good hint."

"Sounds good, but I am worried this is going to get complex and technical. I always hear that the back is very complicated."

"Yes, back pain can be very complex. Many people have had various injuries, including everything from falls to car accidents. What I am going to share with you is not intended to solve the back pain issues for every accident or situation, but rather is a way to have good posture and proper back health to help you and others live pain free."

"I understand. I didn't expect you to fix every back problem out there."

"The good news is that once you start correcting the causes of lower back pain, most of the other postural deficiencies almost take care of themselves.

"That said, have you ever had a sore lower back? Have you ever just moved funny and then you had a shooting pain in your back?"

"Of course I have," replied Timmy. "Who hasn't?"

"Exactly. Lower back pain is probably one of the top forms of musculoskeletal degeneration in the adult population. It is said to affect nearly eight out of ten adults."
http://www.webmd.com/back-pain/default.htm
http://www.medicalnewstoday.com/articles/134732.php
"Wow. I knew it was high, just not that high."

"Yes. So just know that you aren't alone if you've ever experienced lower back pain. I have to admit, I have tweaked my back more than a few times in my life."

"Really? You, who looks like a superhero? You've had back pain?"

"It's true. The good news is that once I started implementing the changes that I am about to teach you, I haven't had a back pain in years. Yes, years!

"Another reason this is so important to me, like you, is that I have family members--aunts, uncles, and grandparents--that have struggled with lower back pain. Two of my relatives ended up in the hospital due to back pain. It hit home for me; these people weren't just statistics, they were my family members!"

Timmy nodded in agreement. "I know I don't look like it, but I am starting to see that we really have some things in common."

"Yes, we do. In fact, both of us have a lot of things in common with most people. Who hasn't had feelings for a family member? Who hasn't wanted to help somebody in need? Who hasn't wanted to improve their own life?"

"Very true," said Timmy.

"Before we get going, let me say that I hate it when people start getting technical when explaining things. I am a big believer in the KISS principle. For our purposes, KISS stands for Keep it Super Simple, and you will hear me reference that a lot. Go ahead and write that in your notes."

Timmy jotted down a few lines in his notebook.

"There will be times when you will want to make things harder than it has to be, and I will tell you to KISS. I have found that in general, life is much easier when you keep it simple."

"I like that a lot!"

"Good. Let's get going.

"If we look at lower back pain in a general sense, there are two main reasons for back pain to occur. One reason is for people in office environments or those that sit for three plus hours per day. The other primary cause is people engaged in long hours of manual labor. One group has back pain due to inactivity, and the other group has pain due to improper overuse, but neither group generally has good posture, which ultimately causes the problems.

"Move over to this chair over here and take a seat. Through a simple demonstration, we are going to examine how the body moves."

Matthew slid a chair around for Timmy.

"That's perfect. Your knees should be bent ninety degrees. Now I want you to take one leg and straighten it at the knee. For that to be possible, the muscles on the front of your thigh contracted, while the muscles on the back of your leg lengthened.

"The muscles on the front of the thigh are called the quadriceps, or quads for short. The muscles on the back of the thigh are called the hamstrings. Both of these muscles had to work together to make your knee extension possible.

"Go ahead and put your foot down. Can you tell me what happened to make that possible?"

"I think I understand this. To lower my leg, the quads had to lengthen, and my hamstrings had to contract."

"That is correct. Does this make sense, Timmy? Do you see how we have a little game of tug-o-war going on?"

"Yes, I see that, but I'm not sure I understand yet how this has anything to do with lower back pain."

"We are getting there.

"When you sit for hours and hours a day, you are doing several things to your body. First, I want you to put your hands on your hips. That area where your fingers are is a muscle group called the hip flexors."

Timmy placed his hands on his hips. "Is this it?"

"Yes, that is it.

"Those are the hip flexors and they are responsible for bringing your knee and thigh up towards your stomach or abdomen. The pivot point is your pelvis.

"The problem arises when you are sitting all day long and these muscles are in a contracted or shortened position for many hours. Like a game of tug-of-war, when one muscle group is contracted, another group has to lengthen to allow that to happen."

"Right, I got that from the original example."

"Great. Let's look deeper as we understand a bit more about the tug-o-war between muscle groups. If the hip flexors are in a contracted or tight position for hours and hours a day, they will have a tendency to keep pulling the pelvis forward, even when you stand up. If the hip flexors are pulling in one direction…"

Timmy interrupted with excitement, "Then there have to be muscles on the other side of that tug-o-war, right?"

"Exactly, you are really catching on!

"Before we get too far, I want you to know that I am making this somewhat simplistic to help you understand. In the human body, the muscles work as groups, so most times there isn't just one muscle pulling on another one. There are multiple muscles pulling in multiple directions. This example allows you to see how one larger muscle group can affect the other groups around it."

"That makes sense. It helps me to understand the concept. Keep going."

"I want you to imagine yourself as a muscle and that you are playing tug-o-war against a stronger opponent. Let's assume you were stretched to the max for hours without getting pulled over the line.

"How you would feel if you were in this position for many hours at a time?"

"I would feel tired and worn out."

"Right, and what do you think would happen if all of a sudden the other 'team' relaxed their grip and you needed to shift gears and start pulling in the other direction? This would equate to a muscle needing to contract."

"Wait a second Matthew, how do you expect me to contract or pull in the other direction? I have been stretched for so long. I am pretty weak and I'm not sure I would be very effective at contracting."

Matthew nodded and smiled.

"That is exactly how your muscles feel when they are placed in an imbalanced state for long periods of time. This means that a muscle that is contracted for a long period of time has a hard time relaxing, and a muscle that has been stretched out for long period of time has a hard time contracting."

"I think this is starting to sink in."

"Good. This happens all over your body with practically every movement. The problem arises when we have poor posture for hours and hours every day, and we repeat those days for weeks, months, years, and even decades in a row.

"Do you see how muscular problems can arise due to these imbalances caused by poor posture, especially with the lower back?"

Timmy nodded in agreement but had a puzzled look on his face. "Is there a way to fix the poor posture caused by these muscle imbalances?"

"Of course there is! We are going to learn to retrain the muscles so we don't have posture problems that can turn into serious issues later on in life."

"Whew, that is a relief to hear."

"Back to those hip flexors. When they are tight from sitting in a contracted position all day, they tend to keep pulling the pelvis forward, even when you stand up. It is hard to keep your back straight if you have tight muscles pulling your pelvis forward and weaker ones trying to keep your pelvis aligned properly."

"Matthew, hold on a second. I get that the tight hip flexors are probably part of the cause of lower back pain, but what does any of this have to do with losing weight?"

"That is a great question, and I am glad you asked!

"Let me ask you a question, Timmy. If you were going to build a very tall building, what is the first thing you would build?"

"Is it the elevator shaft? The plumbing? The roof?"

"That's really easy; I would build the base, or foundation first. You have to have a strong foundation to build upon."

"You are correct.

"Without this strong foundation, there is nothing to support the many floors above it. The body is the same way.

"Let's go back to our tug-o-war example. If your muscles are not in a balanced state due to poor posture, you just can't jump right into exercising or you will probably injure yourself.

"If somebody has poor posture when they are sitting or walking, do you think it is possible for them to have good posture while jogging or running?"

"Let me see if I get this straight. Muscle imbalances due to poor posture and a lack of movement are causing people to move improperly. If somebody walks improperly, which places undue stress on the knees, hips, and back, then you want to correct those issues before moving forward, right?"

"You nailed it! I wouldn't be able to help very many people if they all got injured the first week, now would I?

"I know it seems like a slower road at first, but by establishing a solid foundation, it will allow you to reach your goals faster because you will minimize setbacks due to injury. Not only can an injury be painful, but it will kill your motivation and make it even harder to achieve your goals."

The smile crept back across Timmy's face as the tension flowed out of his body. Just when he was about to get frustrated because Matthew was moving too slowly for his liking, Matthew's well thought-out logic and reasoning proved to have a calming effect.

"Now that you have a better understanding of how the muscles work, let's look at a few of the major changes that are happening to our bodies due to the muscle imbalances caused by poor posture.

"The reason I bring this up is because as I became a certified personal trainer, I really became fascinated with not only looking at other people's posture, but also correcting my own.

"I realized that even though I was in shape, there were things I wasn't doing correctly, and I wanted to minimize or eliminate the chance of injury and pain.

"You see, I have had those 'bent over the sink in the morning' or 'bent down to get something' back pain flare-ups, and they are no fun. I also had a shoulder surgery a few years back, and I realized that if I had done some things differently, I wouldn't have had those problems.

"So that is why I really started looking at posture. I quit seeing what people were wearing, and I started to see how they were standing, sitting, and moving. I would think to myself what they would need to do to correct their posture.

"I would be at the airport or another public place and I often would say to myself, 'That person looks more like they are waddling than walking.'

"Start watching people move when you are out in public. You will see people walking with their feet pointed out to the side, their knees caved inward, and they won't be able to bend their knees properly.

"Timmy, I know this will hit home with you, and I am only bringing it up because I care; there is a reason your shoes are worn the way they are. I know that walking on shoes that are slanted like that can't be comfortable on your feet."

"Matthew, I really want to change," said Timmy with a slight hint of sadness in his voice. "I have known something wasn't right, but I wasn't sure what it was. When I was going to the hospital to see my mom, I actually sat there for a second and looked at my shoes and how they were worn in such a weird angle. I just didn't know what it meant until now."

"That is good. The first thing is that you are aware of the problem, and second, you are motivated to fix it. I have some good news though."

"What's that?"

"I am going to show you in just a few minutes how you can start fixing that issue that is causing your feet and back to hurt today!"

"Really?"

"Yes.

"After years and years of having certain muscles in a stretched out, weak, or underactive state, you can't expect them to all of a sudden work properly. It is like practicing bad habits all week, then trying to do it right during the game on the weekend. It just doesn't work."

"Makes sense to me."

"I have found that when you correct the causes of lower back pain, most of the other posture issues will be corrected as well. How does that sound?"

"That sounds great! What you are about to teach me sounds pretty amazing."

"You know what, it is. But before we start, let's take a five minute break to get some water."

Before Matthew could say anything further, Timmy already had his back to him and was heading out the door.

13

The Secret to Stopping Back Pain

"I'm ready, Matthew; I want to learn that secret stretch you were doing."

"Then let's dive right in!

"As we discussed before, I like to focus on the lower back because it not only affects so many people, but most of the other postural issues stem from lower back issues. Meaning, in the process of correcting lower back issues, I often find that it helps correct other posture issues."

"I like the sound of that."

"Great. I am now going to teach you something I developed called 'The Squeeze.'"

"What is it? A stretch?"

"I like to call it a stretchercise; it is part stretch, but it is also part exercise."

"That sounds pretty cool!"

"It is. The beauty of The Squeeze is that it is something you can do pretty much anytime, anywhere. It is VERY easy, and one of the best things about it is that nobody will know you are doing it! So you don't have to worry about looking weird, or hear comments from people that want to hold you back."

"I like the sound of that. People can be pretty mean when you are overweight, even if you are trying to get into shape."

"During any of the fifty times a day you are standing in line or standing still, or just want to stand up and take a break, do The Squeeze.

"Go ahead and stand up, and I will tell you what to do."
Timmy stood up, ready to follow the instructions.
"Looks good. Here we go.

- Stand 'normal' with your feet shoulder width apart.
- Make sure your toes are pointed forward, with a slight bend in your knees. Your knees should not be locked.
- Now that you are in this position, I want you to squeeze your butt cheeks (glutes) together as hard as you can.
- After that I want you to pull in and tighten your stomach/abs.
- Keep going up your body. Pull your shoulders back, push your chest out, and stand tall.

Hold this position for at least 10 seconds to start. Relax if you want, then tighten everything up again and hold it. You should get to a point where you can hold this position for minutes at a time."

Timmy stood up and noticed that his toes are pointing outward about 30 degrees and not straight ahead. He corrected his feet and then began to tighten his body. His shoulders came back, he pushed his chest out, and his head was held high.

"Looks great. I want you to tell me how you feel."

"I don't know how to explain it, but it is as if the strain off my lower back went away. Plus, I feel like I am three inches taller. It also feels like my waist moved."

"That is great, Timmy! That is how you should feel. I want to take a minute and tell you why your lower back muscles feel better."

"Sounds good, Matthew. I will just keep holding The Squeeze while you talk. It just feels good, plus I can feel my muscles working."

"Great, I am glad you can feel a difference."

"Remember the tug-o-war from earlier? Remember there was the overactive or tight muscle that was pulling, and there was the underactive muscle that was stretched out?"

"Yes."

"Well due to the poor posture most people have, those lower back muscles become overactive and tight and they are trying to do the work that was designed for other muscle groups.

"We have the tight hip flexors pulling the pelvis forward, which causes the glutes and hamstrings to be stretched out.

"Remember how I said that muscles work in groups and that very seldom is it just a tug-o-war between two muscles?"

"Yes, I remember that."

"Well, because the glutes and hamstrings are stretched out, there is another muscle group that starts trying to take up the slack that those two large muscle groups aren't doing.

"Want to guess which muscle?"

"I am going to say the lower back."

"Exactly!

"Now you can see how sitting all day long and having tight hip flexors can end up being a major cause of lower back pain.

"By doing The Squeeze, we are activating the hamstrings and the glutes by contracting and holding them. By contracting these two muscle groups, it is going to force the pelvis from its tilted forward position back to a neutral position.

"I think that is what you meant when you said your 'waist moved.'"

"Yes, that is exactly what I was feeling."

"When the hip flexors relax, and the glutes and hamstrings start doing their job again, the lower back doesn't have to help out, therefore taking the strain off the lower back.

"Here is a diagram that illustrates the anterior pelvic tilt, which we just corrected by doing The Squeeze.

anterior rotation   neutral pelvis

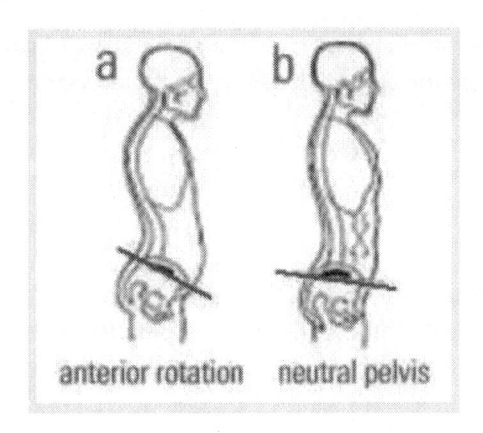

"Anterior means to the front, and you can see in the diagram on the left how the pelvis is tilted forward."

"I see that."

"You can also see how the tight hip flexors would pull that forward, as well as how the back of the pelvis would stretch out the glutes and hamstrings."

"Yes, I see that as well. Amazing how sitting for long periods can throw the body out of such whack."

"Exactly. You see, the glutes are a large, powerful muscle group, but when you sit on them all day and they are in a stretched out position, it is hard for them to get activated again after hours of inactivity.

"The problems get worse over time as the surrounding muscles take over the functions of the weaker muscle. Think of it as a backup system for the muscles of the body. The starting quarterback is out, so we have to bring in this new guy to fill in. Sure, he can run some plays and do the basics, but nowhere near as well as the starter."

Timmy nodded his head while taking it all in.

"When our glutes are weak, the lower back starts acting as the backup quarterback and trying to do part of the job of the glutes. The problem arises when you need to do something that requires all of the lower back muscles, like picking something up.

"They can't do it because they are helping out the glutes and the hamstrings.

"Further problems arise when the 'backup quarterbacks' can't move the body properly. This leads to faulty movement patterns, which change the motion of the body and lead to serious injury."

"Hold on a second. I think something just clicked. So earlier when you said all that stuff about not jumping right into exercising because I might get injured, this is what you were referring to, right?"

"You got it."

"Let me see if I have this straight. By having poor posture, it causes some muscles to be tighter and others to be stretched out and weaker."

"Yes."

"When your body is in that state over a long period of time, the surrounding muscles have to come in to help the weaker muscles like a backup quarterback. When this muscle assisting occurs, two things can happen."

"Keep going."

"First, if a muscle is needed, but it is helping out another, it can lead to injury. This is very common with the lower back because so often it is doing things it isn't designed to do."

"And the second?"

"If you have the surrounding muscles doing the work for weaker muscles long enough, it changes the way in which you move. The body isn't designed to move in such a way, so it usually ends up in injury. How is that?"

"I am very impressed, Timmy. I was a bit worried that I was getting a bit too technical, even though I was trying to keep it simple. I find that once people understand a bit how the body works, it makes it easier for them to see the bigger picture, which I believe you grasped beautifully.

"Does it make sense why I don't want to rush people into exercise without working on that foundation first?"

"Matthew, it really does make sense. By the way, I really like The Squeeze! I have only been doing it for the past several minutes, but I can feel a big difference already. It's weird though, I almost feel more confident."

"Great to hear! Just so you know, that feeling isn't weird at all. By standing tall and adopting good posture, not only will it make you feel more confident, but you will project that confidence to others."

"Makes sense. I have another question though. I can see how The Squeeze helps the lower back, but how does it help some of the other posture issues?"

"Great question.

"The glutes are a very large and important muscle group. When they are not being used, it doesn't just impact the lower back, it also impacts the knees caving inward, and to some extent is part of the reason why the feet turn out.

"Those two things are part of the reason your shoes are wearing out so fast."

"Makes sense."

"When your lower back is in a good place and you are exhibiting good posture, it is very hard to roll your shoulders forward and have your head pushing forward. Those two things would change your posture in such a way that would affect the lower back."

"I see. It makes sense that if you have good posture and take care of your lower back, then most other things fall into place."

"You got it!

"In addition to doing the The Squeeze multiple times throughout your day, just being conscious of your posture will help your back tremendously.

"If you are thinking about your posture, then odds are you are taking action too!

"Here are some quick posture pointers I put together to help with your posture while sitting, driving, or while lifting objects."

Matthew handed him a sheet of paper.

How to Sit Properly at Work:

- Sit up. Keep your back straight and your shoulders back.
- Make sure your butt touches the back of the chair.
- If you are physically able, get one of those chairs where you rest on your shins with no back support.
- It is perfectly ok to use a pillow or special lumbar support to help you maintain the normal curves in your back. I love the Tempur-Pedic lumbar pillow!
- Distribute your body weight evenly on both hips.
- Bend your knees at a right angle keeping your feet flat on the floor. Your knees should be about hip width apart.

- Try to keep your legs straight and not crossed.
- Try to avoid sitting in the same position for more than 30 minutes.
- When at work, you should be sitting close to your computer with the screen tilted up towards you. Adjust your chair height and computer screen so this happens.
- Try keeping your shoulders relaxed by resting your elbows, forearms, and/or arms on your chair or desk.
- When you get more advanced, or if you have a cool work place, sit on an exercise ball. It will work your core and help your posture.
- After sitting for a while; stand up slowly. Take a moment to stretch, and then stand up straight and do The Squeeze exercise we talked about.

While Driving:

- Use a pillow or lumbar support, especially for long trips. Again, I love the Tempur-Pedic lumbar pillow.
- Move the seat close to the steering wheel so that you are sitting up straight and can rest your wrists on the top of the steering wheel.
- This may feel awkward at first, but it is the best position for your posture and safety in case of an accident. From this position, if you are very uncomfortable, you may slide the seat back slightly.
- Your knees should be bent, never locked out, and your feet should be able to reach the pedals.
- A final safety point that doesn't have much to do with posture, but will save you from getting whiplash in the event of an accident, is to raise the headrest so that it is level with your head. Don't keep it pushed down all the way because it looks cool. Set it to a height so that if you get rear-ended, your head will hit the center of the headrest and you won't break your neck.

"I know about this last part because I had a car totaled when I got rear ended several years ago," Matthew explained. When the paramedics arrived, they said I was one out of one hundred that set their headrest correctly, and that is why I had ZERO neck injuries after being rear-ended at approximately forty mph. The impact broke my seat, but because my headrest was set properly, I did not get whiplash and wasn't hurt."

How to lift objects properly:

- Before you lift a heavy object, have a plan of what you are going to do with the object once you pick it up. Do The Squeeze while you are thinking about it.
- Once you have a plan, take a wide stance and plant your feet close to the object you are going to pick up. Tighten your stomach muscles and lift the object using your leg muscles. Bend at your knees and hips and keep your back straight.
- NEVER bend over at the waist or keep your knees locked!
- Move in a fluid motion; do not try to jerk the object off the floor.
- Hold heavy objects close to your body. Always keep your stomach (core) muscles tight. Don't arch your back.
- To set down the object, plant your feet in a wide stance. Tighten your abs (core), and bend at the hips and knees to set the object.

"Thanks, Matthew. Between this list of pointers and The Squeeze, I will definitely be working on this. I can't stand the way my shoes wear out so quickly, plus it hurts my feet."

"It takes most people two to four weeks to break and change a habit. That is why we are starting here.

"If you take one month and focus on your posture, not only will you have gone a long way towards changing your habits, but also you will have established a foundation where we should be able to increase your activity levels and get your body moving properly and injury free.

"We will cover this more in a following session, but while you are taking this month to work on your posture, you will simultaneously be adopting solid nutritional habits.

"This means after one month, you will have changed your posture and eating habits, which is a huge step towards living The Lean Life!"

"Wow, you really thought this through, Matthew. So let me get this straight. It takes about a month to change and create a new habit. I am going to take this first month to work on my posture and at the same time it sounds like you will be helping me making some changes to the way I eat. That way, after a month I will have good posture habits, as well as start to have better eating habits."

"Bingo."

"Even though it doesn't sound like I will be exercising yet, I have to assume that I will probably start losing weight just by doing The Squeeze and eating better."

"Yes, you will start losing weight because of those two things, but we are definitely going to get you moving more as well. There is definitely a plan, as too much too soon usually ends in burn out, and that is where we end up injured or get the 'yo-yo' dieting effect because we were trying to do too much too soon.

"Again, everything I am teaching you is about a lifestyle. It is something you can do for the rest of your life, not just a week or a month or a year. The goal is to make these habits part of your life, and you are well on your way.

"Let's take a break and meet back here in forty-five minutes."

"Sounds good to me! I think I am actually going to walk to the cafeteria, get some food, and come back."

"Enjoy your lunch, Timmy. See you back here in a bit."

14

Just MOVE! A Little Goes a Long Way

"Welcome back! Not only did you make it back within the forty-five minutes, but it looks like you broke a little sweat," Matthew said, greeting Timmy on his way back from the cafeteria.

"Whew, I haven't walked that far in a long time. I have to say, it felt really good though. I did notice that I really have to think about keeping my feet straight. I know it is going to take some work to correct it, but I really think my worn shoes aren't helping any."

"You are correct on all accounts! It is going to take some time to retrain the body, but I think a new pair of shoes is definitely in order. I used to have a similar problem, so I know that when the soles of your shoes get that slanted, it can make things worse.

"I am very proud of you for walking to the cafeteria and back. I know that was a big step for you! It is also good because it rolls right into the next topic I want to talk with you about.

"Remember our 'crisis in movement' discussion and how our lack of motion as a country is largely responsible for our obesity problem?"

"Yes, I remember that."

"I don't know if you saw it or not, but *USA Today* just published an article saying that America has the highest rate of obesity out of thirty-three countries with advanced economies (http://www.usatoday.com/news/health/weightloss/2010-09-24-fatusa24_ST_N.htm)."

"Wow."

"Yes. There are many factors, but I believe a big one is our prosperity as a country where everybody has a car and/or access to public transportation.

"The downside to having this access to transportation is that as a whole, nobody is walking anymore. Walking is excellent exercise, and it contributes to muscular as well as cardiovascular health."

"You are totally right, Matthew. Up until today, I would always use the campus shuttle to get around instead of walking. It never crossed my mind to walk ten or more minutes to get anywhere. Even back at home, we would drive everywhere and always park as close to the door as possible."

"You are certainly not alone. Earlier today, we discussed how most people were becoming obese by the slow and steady gaining of one to two pounds per month over an extended period of time. Nobody notices the pound or two gained in a month, but everybody notices the effects of putting on fifteen to thirty pounds over a year. Sure, part of that is due to nutrition, but if people just walked a few minutes per day, they could completely wipe out and even reverse the trend of gaining a pound per month.

"I am not saying that everybody needs to go for thirty to forty-five minute power walks each day, even though that would be great if they did. What I am trying to do is just to get you and everybody else to be aware of the benefits of just moving!"

"Wow, it is pretty amazing how the little things can make such a big difference," said Timmy. "I have never thought about things in this way. I just look back over the past ten years and think that if I had just walked a bit more each day, I wouldn't be where I am today."

"That's right, Timmy! We will get into this in a little bit more depth here soon, but I am going to show you the long-term impact of your walk to the cafeteria and back."

"I can't wait to see that."

"What I want you to understand is that it doesn't take being a workout junkie to lose weight. Sure, it will happen faster if you do workout, but let's be honest, most people don't want to and aren't going to stick with a workout program. They might for a bit, but they will go back to their old habits and the weight will return. I want you to see that little things make a big difference over time.

"Doesn't mean you have to set aside time to 'go for a walk' to reap the benefits, either. Just making an effort to walk more during your day-to-day routine will go a long way. Just like you did at lunch!"

Timmy smiled.

"The next time you are running errands, I want you to park towards the middle or back of the parking lot and walk to the store. It might seem like a little thing, but over the course of a year that equates to losing several pounds of body fat!"

"Really? Are you sure?"

"Yes, I am. I don't count calories and we don't count calories as part of The Lean Life program, but I want to show you the effect of adding a few more 'steps' to your day. To do this, we need a unit of measurement, which will be the calorie.

"Before we get started, I want you to know that determining the calories burned in an activity can vary widely depending on the size and makeup of the individual, as well as the intensity of the exercise, so just use these numbers as a guide.

"For the purpose of this example, we will give a range for people weighing from approximately 150 to 180 pounds. Assuming the same intensity, if you are 150-160 pounds, you will be towards the lower end of the range. If you are 170-180 pounds, you will be towards the higher end.

"If you are, say, 250 to 300 pounds or more, just know that you will be burning even more calories.

"Again, the point isn't to count calories. This is an example of how the 'little things' make a big difference over time!

"For an hour of moderate walking, you will burn about 230-270 calories. Let's take that hour and split it up by six days. That breaks down to ten minutes of walking per day.

"If you parked at the back of the parking lot and walked into work or school, that would take, say, three to five minutes, maybe more, maybe less. Then another three to five minutes at the end of the day. Right there you already have six to ten minutes of extra walking during your day, and you didn't even go to your car at lunch or run any errands.

"For the sake of this example, let's just assume you did the bare minimum and got your ten minutes of extra walking in each day. Let's also use a round number in the middle and say you burned 250 calories per hour.

"An extra 250 calories burned over those six days translates into burning an extra 1250 calories during each thirty day month just by parking farther out and walking into work, school, or into the store.

"1250 calories per month times twelve months is 15,000 calories over the course of a year!"

"That sounds nice, but what does that really mean?"

"There are 3500 calories in a pound of fat. So just by walking further into work or the store each day, you can burn over four pounds of body fat by doing a bare minimum of walking."

"Wow, just think how many calories I am burning when I have to walk ten to fifteen minutes to get anywhere on campus."

"That's right, Timmy. You can literally walk your pounds away. It doesn't require going to the gym or any other drastic changes to your life. A little bit of effort goes a long way!

"For most people, if they had done this one simple thing with zero other changes over the past five years, they would probably be eighteen to twenty pounds lighter.

"Do you see how these little things can make a big difference and turn things around for you, your family, and the obesity epidemic as a whole?"

Shaking his head in a state of disbelief, "I just can't believe it. I always thought you had to get yelled at by a personal trainer and go through periods of intense pain where people actually throw-up and cry like on the weight-loss TV shows. It is so refreshing to see there is another way. I can walk without fear of injury, and I don't mind doing it."

"That is what The Lean Life is all about, Timmy! Making those easy, barely noticeable changes that will have a big payoff over time.

"Let's get really crazy and take things a step further. What would happen over the course of the year if you took the stairs instead of the elevator or escalator?"

Out of the corner of his eye, Matthew saw Timmy's lip quiver.

"I know what you are thinking; 'stairs suck, I hate taking the stairs.'"

"Yup. At my weight, taking the stairs is a monumental task," replied Timmy.

"I hear you, I really do. I know it is hard to carry that extra weight up the stairs, and even harder on the joints when coming down. But, it is something we are going to work towards. The good news is that as you start losing weight, it will only get easier.

"Stairs are good for you because they not only work the cardiovascular system, but they are great for working and toning the leg muscles.

"I am not saying that if you work in a skyscraper or other high rise to take the stairs twenty flights, but if you are in a building that is six stories or less, you should seriously think about taking the stairs more times than not. Use it as a goal and something to work towards."

"I'm glad I am only on the second floor. One flight of stairs is enough!"

"That is perfect. Start with only taking one to three flights of stairs, and work up from there. Every little bit helps. Say you take the stairs to the third floor and then get on the elevator to go the rest of the way. Those little challenges will not only help you physically, but more importantly, they will keep you mentally focused on your goal of losing weight!

"Here is another example. A 150-pound individual will burn about ten calories per minute going up, and seven calories per minute going down the stairs. If you work on the second or third story of a building, you can easily burn twenty to forty calories each time you make a trip up and back down the stairs.

"If you take the stairs only two times per day, you can easily burn another fifty calories per day. Try doing this behavior five days a week and you have burned another 250 calories per week, or 1000 calories per month!

"1000 calories per month times twelve months is 12,000 calories and over three pounds of body fat.

"So just by walking further into work and taking the stairs, you can burn enough calories to lose seven pounds of body fat in a year without even trying!"

"Wait a second. So you are telling me that if I had just moved a little bit more over the past ten plus years, I could be seventy pounds lighter?" enquired Timmy.

"I hate to say it, but yes. With no change to your diet and just moving more in your daily life, you could easily be seventy pounds lighter over that time period."

A look of sadness and regret crossed Timmy's face.

"What's done is done. Neither of us can go back in time and change the past, but what we can do is change our habits in the present and live for a bright future," exclaimed an energetic Matthew.

"Just think, that example we used is only on the stairs at your work, but it doesn't include all the malls, airports, and other public places where you can take the stairs over the escalator."

"What if they don't have stairs, just an escalator?"

"What about it? Just because the stairs or sidewalks are moving, doesn't mean you don't have to. It is ok to walk up a moving escalator, just be careful when you step off. The same applies to moving sidewalks at airports; get on and walk!"

Timmy just smiled. "I get it. When in doubt, move!"

"Precisely! Let's take a look at your accomplishment during lunch. You walked to the cafeteria, ate lunch, and walked back in about forty-five minutes. You estimated that it took you twelve to fifteen minutes to walk there each way. For the sake of using round numbers, let's just say it took you fifteen minutes each way. So you walked for thirty minutes just at lunch."

Timmy nodded intently.

"I don't know exactly how many calories you are burning, but it is easy to say it is at the higher end of the range. So let's just assume you burn 300 calories an hour walking, and you just walked for half an hour, so that is 150 calories.

"Let's assume you walk to the cafeteria just one time per day, seven days a week. That means you will walk for three-and-a-half hours. That is going to equate to 1050 extra calories burned per week, which is 4200 calories per month."

"I see where you are going with this. If I don't change any other habits, but I just walk to go eat once per day, I will lose over a pound a month right there."

"You nailed it."

"Let me guess, you are probably going to show me some other little changes that I can make that will have a similar effect. So if I make several small changes, I should be able to lose two to five pounds per month without any big changes, if that is the way I want to go."

"That is it, Timmy. I am not trying to make people do anything drastic. I can't do that, and besides, it won't work. I can't make you want it. If you want more, I can give more, but the purpose of The Lean Life is to show people they can lose weight and get where they want to be by making small changes over time, thus leading to a lifestyle that keeps you lean long-term."

"I understand. I wasn't thinking about myself so much as I was a member of my family. I am motivated to learn and turn my life around. I am prepared to do the extra work, but like you said, many people just want it to be 'easy' and don't want big change. That is why I like what you are telling me. Even little changes over time can make a big difference!"

"That's it! The little things add up over time! Look at how easy something as simple as just walking a little bit and taking the stairs can impact your waistline over the course of the year.

"I also understand how an overweight person like yourself can look at the situation and think there is no way they can lose the weight. I know it can seem like an insurmountable task. I know you see shows like *The Biggest Loser* and you think if it takes yelling, puking, and being miserable to lose weight, you don't want any part of it.

"I get it. Very few people would, and that is why I think we need something that speaks to more people like you. Sure, it isn't going to happen overnight, but you can turn things around and be at a normal weight in several months to a few years for the heaviest people."

"You really think I could be at a normal weight in only a few years?"

"Yes, I do. I have one friend that lost 167 pounds in two years. And another that lost over 100 pounds in about 18 months. That really isn't very much time, both of them did it safely, and they both kept the weight off."

"Wow, impressive!"

"Yes, it is.

"The beauty of it is that once the weight starts to come off, things start to snowball, in a good way. Many people start to work out and eat better to speed things along as they start seeing results, which is what I love to see--people taking control of their lives because they want to, not because a doctor or somebody else forced them."

Timmy nodded his head.

"I know we have spent quite a bit of time talking already today, but I know you still have some time until your class later this afternoon. I have two more things I want to cover today, and from there I think you will have a good foundation of things to start working on.

"Do you want to take a short break and power through the last two things?"

"Sure, that sounds great. I want to do The Squeeze, get some water, and walk around a bit to stretch my legs."

"Sounds like a plan to me. Let's meet back here in ten minutes."

15

Increase Your Metabolism by 3%

"Hey Matthew, can I ask you something?" inquired Timmy.

"Sure, what is it?"

"I know it has only been a few hours, but am I crazy to think that I already feel better and different? I mean, on one hand, I really haven't done that much compared to what you probably do on a normal day. But on the other hand, walking for forty-five minutes today, eating less, and standing up straight is so different than anything I have done in many years. I really do feel different!"

"First off, you aren't crazy. This has been a big day for you. You have walked more today than you probably have in the past week or so combined. I think people forget how nice it is to be out walking in the fresh air. Not to mention that you ate less, drank more water, and started working on your posture. I would say that is a big success and you should feel good!"

"I do feel good, but I also know you probably do more on a given day than I do."

"It doesn't matter. I don't want you comparing yourself to me or to other people. All that matters is what you accomplish, and that you are enjoying your new Lean lifestyle and making it work for you."

"I think I understand. Just because somebody else ran for an hour, it doesn't make my forty-five minutes of walking any less of an accomplishment. It doesn't matter what somebody else does, I just need to focus on what I am doing, work my plan, and I will get where I want to go."

"Exactly! Work your plan, not somebody else's plan. I am so happy you are getting this. Your family is going to be lucky to have you as their coach.

"Let's move on, as I want to teach you about the lifeblood of your body."

"What is that?"

"If I told you there was an EASY way to increase your metabolism by 3%, would you do it? This means that your body would burn 3% more calories every day, even while you are at rest."

"Are you kidding me, who wouldn't want to boost their metabolism 3% and burn those extra calories with no effort? Of course I would! What do I need to do?" enquired a perked up Timmy.

"I will get to the specifics in a minute, but this is an easy one to do."

"What is it?"

"You need to drink water."

"Water, really? That's it?"

"So simple, yet so few people do it.

"Water should be your drink of choice throughout the day as it is very crucial for weight loss and optimal health. Studies show that about 75% of the people in America are chronically dehydrated. If you are even mildly dehydrated, which means a water loss of only one or two percent, your metabolism can slow about three percent!"

"So you are telling me that by drinking enough water, I can get my metabolism fired up and running on all cylinders?"

"Yes. Not only that, but if you switch from drinking just one can of soda or fruit juice per day to water, that alone will save you almost fifteen pounds of body fat per year!"

"Really?"

"Yes. One can of regular soda or juice has about 200 calories. Two hundred calories only five days per week is 1000 calories a week. Fifty-two weeks in a year means 52,000 calories saved, which divided by 3500 calories in a pound of fat means a saving of 14.8 pounds per year!"

"Wow. I can see how this really adds up. Drinking water in place of soda, a bit of walking and taking the stairs, and you are already at twenty-five pounds a year lost!"

"See how little things over time make a BIG difference?"

"Yes, I do."

"Aside from that, the human body is comprised of about 70% water. Believe it or not, you can go weeks without food, but only days without water. Water is crucial for removing toxins and waste from your body, not to mention it is the lifeblood of your body. Your skin, heart, and muscles all depend on having enough water to by hydrated so they can perform at their best."

"How much water do you drink per day, Matthew?"

"I try to drink at least a gallon per day. Some people drink eight, eight ounce glasses of water per day. Some say to drink half of your bodyweight in ounces If you weigh 200 pounds, drink 100oz of water. I think any of those are fine. The main thing is that your urine should never be dark yellow and you shouldn't be thirsty."

"Ok. Good to know. I will shoot for that gallon of water per day."

"That is a good start. There is another very important reason overweight people should drink lots of water if they are intent on losing weight."

"What's that?"

"Their skin looks healthier and it can minimize stretch marks. Drinking plenty water will help the elasticity of the skin as their bodies begin to shrink. If you lose weight too fast, you will have lots of extra skin hanging around. If you lose the weight in a steady manner and drink lots of water, you can minimize stretch marks and hopefully have your skin shrink along with your body."

"I never thought about that."

"Most people don't until it is too late. Drinking plenty of water will only help you during your quest to lose weight in a healthy manner."

"So being dehydrated is definitely not a good thing then."

"Not at all. Not only can being dehydrated slow your metabolism, but dehydration can also mask itself as hunger. That could be a double whammy if you are trying to lose weight. You are eating more calories because you think you are hungry, but in actuality your body is just dehydrated.

"So you are consuming more calories when your body's metabolism is actually slowing down. Not exactly the best recipe for weight loss!"

"Ouch. That stinks, but it does make sense. There have been times when I thought I was super hungry, but for some reason I ended up chugging water or juice and I didn't feel hungry anymore."

"Wait, you chugged water or juice, which one was it?"

"Ok, you got me, it was usually juice," replied Timmy, like a kid caught in a little white lie.

"I know, I know. Water doesn't taste good, or it doesn't have any taste, but it is the best thing for you, especially if you want to lose body fat.

"Well, guess what, I have several things you can do to not only make the water taste better by adding some flavor, but also make it healthy for your body too!"

"Cool, what are they?"

"My three favorite ways to add flavor and spice up my water are as follows:

"- I like to make a lot of all natural green tea. I will take ten to fifteen tea bags and make a huge pitcher of tea to leave in my refrigerator, and then drink it for several days, or all in one day in some cases. I do not add any sweetener to the tea, natural or otherwise.

"- I love to add lemon to my water. I typically use fresh lemons, which are the best, but I have used Real Lemon juice from the bottle as well. I will put a few slices of lemon in or just squirt some of the Real Lemon juice into my glass or water bottle and go. I don't add any sugar or artificial sweetener; just water, ice, and lemon juice.

"- Lastly, I will add cucumber to my water. Again, this is pretty easy, and there are two ways you can do it. You can do the pitcher in the fridge full of the cucumber slices, or you can add cucumber slices to your individual glass or water bottle.

"When I am on the go, lemon water is probably the easiest to do and what I default to most of the time. It is so easy to keep lemon slices in the fridge or squirt some Real Limon into my water bottle."

"My mom likes to drink Diet Coke and make a lot of Crystal Light because it had five calories or no calories, I forget. Is that ok?"

"I know a lot of people, like your mom, like to add Crystal Light and other low/no-calorie powders to their water. My advice is to use those with moderation. The reason they have 'no calories' is because they are loaded with artificial sweeteners.

"My advice on artificial sweeteners is this: avoid them as much as possible. I am not going to go into too much depth right now, as that is a topic for another day. Just know there is a lot of debate about the various artificial sweeteners and the long-term effects they have on the body. Again, moderation is the key. Here are the big four artificial sweeteners:

- **Sucralose (Splenda)**
- **Aspartame (Equal)**
- **Saccharine (Sweet'N Low)**
- **Acesulfame Potassium (aka - acesulfame K or ace-K)**"

"My advice is to look for the all-natural sweeteners Stevia or Xylitol. There are several brand names for those two sweeteners."

"So you are saying that even the zero calorie diet sodas aren't healthy either? My mom drinks Diet Coke like it is going out of style," said a perplexed Timmy.

"A lot of people drink diet sodas to avoid all of the sugar and calories in the real sodas. The problem is that a lot of people are drinking three to six diet sodas per day, and there is still debate on the long-term effects of some of the artificial sweeteners.

"Having diet soda or even regular soda every now and then is fine. Enjoy it. The best thing to do is to make your lifestyle something that doesn't revolve around any type of soda. Make soda a treat, a reward, or something for the weekends."

"Sounds like a good idea, but that is going to be tough for me."

"Trust me, I know it is tough. I didn't drink much soda as a kid, but I always loved carbonation. When I was on my own, I used to go to the store and buy four to five different 12-packs of diet sodas to stock my fridge. I drank one and occasionally two diet sodas per day. I had the diet versions of Sunkist, Mountain Dew, Cherry Coke, Vanilla Coke, Vanilla Pepsi, Dr. Pepper, and Cherry Vanilla Dr. Pepper. You name it, I probably had it in my fridge at one point or another."

"That is funny. I can't believe you were a soda person, Matthew."

"I know. Then I started reading more about the artificial sweetener aspartame and its effects on the body. I didn't know exactly what to believe, so over two years ago I took a 90-day 'aspartame challenge' where I was to eliminate aspartame from my diet. I have to tell you, after the first week, I didn't miss it one bit. At first it was hard because aspartame is in all of that low/no-calories stuff like diet sodas, sugar-free Jello, and Crystal Light, just to name a few."

"So what did you drink?"

"I switched from sodas to natural flavored sparkling waters and I haven't looked back. Sure, I still have an occasional soda--I love my Diet Mountain Dew--but I have to tell you that after ditching the artificial sweeteners, when I do go back and have a diet soda, the taste is really noticeable.

"When you do decide to kick artificial sweeteners out of your daily life, go several months without them; you will notice how they have a 'chemical' taste to them. Personally, I prefer the natural flavors to the 'chemical' or 'artificial' ones."

Timmy seemed almost sad at the news that Matthew doesn't drink much soda anymore.

"Don't worry, Timmy; I am not going to take away your soda without giving you a tasty alternative!"

"Good thing!"

"Take Perrier, or other sparkling or soda water, and mix POM or other pomegranate juice with it. Sure, pomegranate has sugar in it, but it is natural sugar from fruit, and besides, you are diluting it. I will usually do like eighty percent water and twenty percent pomegranate. Start there and see how your taste buds like it. Sometimes I will only do a splash of the POM, and it still tastes great and gives the drink a nice red color."

"Sounds pretty tasty there, Matthew."

"You bet it is.

"If you do feel the need to sweeten your water, tea, or coffee, I suggest using Stevia as it is an all-natural, low-calorie sweetener. I suggest using the natural sweeteners and flavoring to make the transition to drinking water easier.

"I know it sounds hard at first, but just trust me, after a week or so without it, you really won't miss it at all.

"If you can make the change to drinking water in place of sugar-rich juices and sodas, you will feel better, have more energy, and burn a lot more body fat. So give it a try. What have you got to lose except for a few pounds?"

"I have to admit. After all the walking I did today, nothing felt better than the cold water out of the water fountain," exclaimed Timmy.

"Isn't it funny how it all works? You start walking more and your body automatically wants water, and not just that, but *you* want it as well. It has only been half a day for you, Timmy, and you are already feeling a difference. Just wait until you get past that three-week mark and these good habits become part of your new Lean lifestyle. You are going to be a different person here soon!"

"I am looking forward to it, but more importantly, I can't wait to share what I have learned with my mom and the rest of my family. When I tell them that making a few easy changes will make a big difference, and they see the change in me, I know they will follow."

"That's great, Timmy. Let's take a quick break so that we can cover the final topic of today. After that, I think you will have a good foundation to build upon.

"Take five minutes and I will meet you back right here."

"Sounds good," replied an upbeat Timmy.

16

Salad Plates, Kiddie Bowls and Portion Control

"Before we get going on our last topic today, I want you to know it is a pleasure working with you. I can truly see you want to change your life and are engaged with our conversation. There is nothing better than working with somebody like yourself who wants to learn and bring positive change to your life," Matthew said encouragingly. "I have no doubt in my mind that you will get where you want to go."

"Me either, Matthew. I have never really had good role models in my life. Talking with you and John makes me feel awesome, and it has opened my eyes to so many things. I always thought I was stuck being 'bigger' because that is what Mom used to say, but now I realize that isn't the case."

"You got that right!

"It is up to you. If you decide to make some or all of the small changes we have talked about today and stick with them, you will see results.

"That said, I want to talk about one last thing today, then you can head off to your late afternoon class.

"I want to show you something you can do today that will automatically help you eat less and lose weight, WITHOUT making you feel deprived.

"You will find this pretty funny--heck, many of my friends do, and they let me know about it."

Matthew reached into the bag by his desk and pulled out a small, clear, plastic bowl.

"I don't even know where or how I acquired this bowl, and I am almost embarrassed to say this, but I have used that bowl pretty much every day for the past ten years."

"Go ahead, let it out. I can see that you are about to explode."

Timmy's whole body was shaking he was laughing so hard. "You eat out of that tiny little thing? That is hilarious! Not only that, but you have kept that small crappy bowl for a decade!"

"Yes, I know it is bad. And yes, I only have that one bowl, not a set of them."

Timmy wiped his eyes as his laughter died down.

"Now that your laughing has subsided, why do you think I like that bowl so much?"

"I have no idea," said Timmy laughing out loud again.

"Let me tell you.

"Yes, it is a cute little indestructible bowl, but the real reason why I like it is its size."

"So it's tiny. Why would you keep it for that reason?"

"I use this bowl for cereal, ice cream, soups, and more. The reason I like it has to do with portion control!"

"Portion control? What's that?"

"Let me show you. Which bowl would you rather eat from?" Matthew pulled a regular bowl from his bag and placed it side by side with his plastic bowl on the table in front of them.

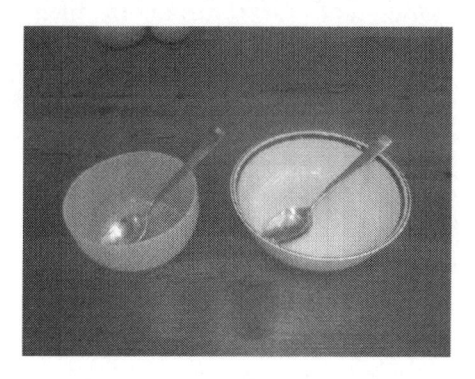

"Well, duh, I would take bigger bowl."

"I know, most people would. The thing is, when you put a standard ¾ or 1 cup serving of cereal in each bowl, one bowl appears to have a lot more food in it, as the other bowl barely has the bottom covered up."

Timmy looked up at Matthew.

"I can see that, because the clear bowl is a lot smaller."

"Exactly. In the other bowl, it takes two to three servings of cereal to make it look full.

"I have done a similar test with friends. I give them a typical cereal bowl and a box of cereal, and tell them to pour a bowl like they would for breakfast."

Matthew slammed his fist on the desk.

"Then I tackle them before they have a chance to add milk!"

Timmy jumped out of his seat.

"Just kidding! You should have seen the look on your face," said Matthew with a good laugh.

"I politely tell them to stop as I get out my measuring cups to see exactly how many servings they poured in their bowl."

"Really?"

"Yes, it is deceiving to most people. They look at most cereals as being pretty light and healthy and not loaded with calories, but the issue is that they have no idea of the serving size.

"Often what I have found is that using a standard cereal bowl, people will pour two to three times the serving size into their bowl.

"I have seen many people read the side of the box and go, 'Cool, only 180 calories,' and start pouring into their bowl. What they don't realize is that they poured in the amount of three servings! Those 180 calories on the box turned into 540 calories in their bowl because they were not aware of the serving size.

"Here is the deal; the brain doesn't register serving sizes. All it sees is a lot of empty space, and that doesn't 'look' satisfying."

"I get it. The smaller bowl looks fuller with less food, so automatically the brain 'feels' a sense of satisfaction."

"Yes, and the same thing applies to your plates. I use salad plates for most of my meals as 'regular' plates are so big, especially nowadays, that even when you put large portions of food on them, it doesn't look 'filling' to the brain because there is so much open space left on the plate.

"I definitely know my portion sizes, but there are times when I am eating at a friend's house, I put the food on my plate, and it just doesn't look like enough, but I know that it is more food than I normally eat. The only reason I catch myself is because I am very aware of what constitutes a correct portion size."

"Hey Matthew, what is a correct portion size?"

"We will cover this in depth later, but a good rule of thumb for meats is that they should be about the size of the palm of your hand, minus the fingers. For fruits and veggies, about the size of your fist; and for potatoes or rice, a little bit smaller than the palm of your hand.

"Even without knowing what the exact portion sizes are, by just eating on smaller plates and bowls, your mind will help tell you that it is 'enough' food.

"I use the little bowl for my cereal and desserts and salad plates for most of my other meals. Make the switch to smaller plates and bowls and you too will slowly start to see those pounds that crept on over the past few months or years start sliding away."

"I don't know, Matthew. Doesn't look like those bowls or plates are very big."

"Trust me, you won't feel like you are depriving yourself. In actuality, because your smaller plate or bowl will look 'fuller,' your brain won't know the difference.

"Make the change to smaller plates and bowls and you won't be disappointed at the results. Again, like all of the other habits that we are changing, this one is going to take the same two weeks to a month to become ingrained. How does that sound?"

"It sounds really good! I don't mean to cut us short, but we need to start wrapping things up so I can walk to my next class. I need to give myself enough time so I won't be late," said an upbeat Timmy.

"Won't be an issue at all, as I was about finished anyway. The last thing I want to do is recap the main things we learned today."

"I got it, I got it!" exclaimed Timmy.

"I am going to work on the following four main points. First, I am going to work on my posture by doing The Squeeze throughout the day. Second, I am going to 'move' more by walking to class and just walking more in general. Third, I am going to drink water in place of sodas and juice. And finally, I am going to use smaller bowls and salad plates when I eat!"

"You nailed it, Timmy! If you commit to just doing those four small things…"

"I know, I know. Little things over time will make a BIG difference!"

"I can't believe how much you have changed over just the past few hours. It is like you are a new person. You are standing taller and it seems like you have a new mindset and outlook on life."

"You know, Matthew, thanks to you I do. I always thought that I was just 'stuck' this way, and that this is the way God made me. After all, that is what my mom told me for years. You let me see that that isn't the case. I can't wait to let my mom and the rest of the family know what I have learned."

"Like I told you earlier, you are going to be able to help a lot of people. I am glad you are feeling good right now, but just know that you are going to have moments where self-doubt and old habits pop up. When those doubts arise, I want you to be strong and not revert back to the bad habits of your past.

"I want you to know you can reach out to me if something comes up and you need somebody to talk to. I don't do this for very many people, but here is a card with my cell phone number and email on it. Don't hesitate to call me. I want you to succeed!"

"I know you do, Matthew. But more importantly, you don't know how bad I want this. I do not want to end up in the hospital because of a heart attack, and I know that is in my future if I don't turn things around now," said Timmy with a serious tone in his voice.

"Stick with those four things for the month and you will have a new set of healthy habits for the rest of your life. I don't think you will have to worry about hospitals or heart attacks if you do.

"You are still very young, Timmy, and besides, it is never too late to turn things around. You can tell your mom and dad I said that, as I know that it can be tougher for older people to see that it isn't too late to start a healthy lifestyle.

"Anyway Timmy, you had better get to class. I hope you still have some blank paper after all of the notes you took. I will see you next Wednesday, and remember, don't hesitate to call or email me if you have questions along the way."

"Thanks Matthew, I will see you next week!"

Timmy left the office and headed off to class.

A few moments later, John pokes his head in to the office.

"Hey Matthew, how did things go with Timmy? I saw him on his way out, and he had a big smile on his face and what looked like some pep in his step."

"Things went very well, John. I gave him four little things to work on. If he does those things, he will get where he wants to go. I feel very good about him."

"What do you think will happen if he 'stumbles,' so to speak?" inquired John.

"Honestly, I don't think it will shake him very much. He gets it. The motivation of seeing what happened to his mother and knowing he was headed down the same path will keep him on track.

"Another thing is that I start simple with people. I start with a few easy things they can do that are not big changes. They will start seeing results, and then they will want to know and do more. You can't force it."

"Very true, Matthew."

"Sure, if he started working out two hours a day and eating perfectly, it could happen faster, but that isn't realistic. Takes time to get to that point.

"My gut feeling is that Timmy will want to know more, in due time. I am excited to watch his progress, but more importantly, I am excited to see how he influences others. He doesn't know it yet, but he is going to be an inspiration to many people."

"You are right, Matthew. I learn something every time I talk with you. For somebody with your appearance, you really do have a heart and want to help people. I just don't think enough people get to see that side of you. I am really glad that you are able to work with Timmy. Even though I was heavy once, I certainly don't know enough to help him with his health and weight issues."

"Thank you for the compliment, John. You might not know what to recommend as far as health and fitness goes, but you know a lot about helping people's mindset and that is the most important thing of all. Without the right mindset, no weight loss or self-improvement is possible. Working on Timmy's mindset, confidence, and attitude will have such a huge impact on his life, and work hand in hand with his weight loss.

"Not to mention that it does help that you were heavy once and can share your experience with him.

"I hate to cut our conversation short, John, but I have to run to another appointment. Have a great day and good luck on your Monday meeting with Timmy!"

"Thanks, Matthew! You have a great afternoon as well, and I will see you later on."

They both left the office and parted ways.

17

Letter to Mom #2

Wednesday, September 15

Dear Mom,

I would ask how you are doing, but I know you have to be doing great! I hope you are following the doctor's orders by getting plenty of rest and improving your habits. I know it isn't going to be easy, but just think about playing with Jessica's kids when she has them someday. She is going to want her children to play with their grandma!

I know how you love to worry about me, but just know I am doing great! Lots of good things are happening to me. Remember when I told you about John, the counselor that reminds me of Uncle David, and how he had a surprise for me? Well, he had a surprise all right!

He introduced me to this guy that looks like a pro athlete or cartoon superhero. I'm serious! He is a personal trainer named Matthew, and you can see this guy's muscles through his clothes. He is super fit, and he really knows his stuff, but most importantly, he is taking me under his wing and teaching me how to be healthy and lose weight. The really neat thing is how he makes it so simple!

I have to be honest with you, I was really scared when you were in the hospital. I was scared for you, but I got really scared for myself when I was trying to find you in the hospital. I didn't tell you, but some lady asked me if I was there for the "High Risk Health" meeting or something like that. I assume she stopped me because I was overweight. There is more. I was so out of breath from walking, I had to stop and sit down. I am too young to feel like this, and if I don't change, I will end up having a heart attack like you and that scares me.

I spent a few hours with Matthew today, and I learned so many things. I learned that I didn't gain weight overnight, but over time, and most importantly, that I don't have to be overweight anymore. I don't want you to have another heart attack either. I want you and the whole family to be healthy.

You won't believe this Mom, but I walked to the cafeteria and to class today. I didn't take the shuttle once! Matthew said I should "just move," which means walking more. It was super hard, but I walked for almost an hour today, not at once, but over the entire day. We talked about four little things that I can do to start peeling off the pounds, and walking more was the first one.

When I would get to where I was going, I was so thirsty, so I just drank water like Matthew does. Not only is it good for your body, but I learned most people are chronically dehydrated and by drinking water you can raise your metabolism by 3%! Drinking water is an easy way to burn more calories, and it is one of the four topics we discussed.

There is one thing I didn't think I was going to like, but Matthew was right, I didn't even notice. He said I should eat my meals on salad plates instead of dinner plates. The brain sees a full plate as satisfying; it doesn't care how big the plate is. You can take the same amount of food and put it on the dinner plate, and the brain will tell you to add food to the plate because there is a lot of empty space.

I have been doing this for lunch and dinner, and it makes a big difference. I am totally tricking my brain. I don't feel hungry, and I thought I would!

The fourth thing I learned was this awesome thing Matthew calls a stretchercise. It is a stretch and an exercise. The cool thing about it is that you can do it anywhere, and get this Mom, nobody can tell you are doing it!

Here is what you do: stand normal with your feet shoulder width apart. Make sure your toes are pointed forward. Now squeeze your butt cheeks together (yeah Mom, I said butt cheeks!). Now squeeze your stomach muscles (otherwise known as your abdominals or abs). While holding this, pull your shoulders back and keep your head high. Just hold this for 10 seconds, then relax. Work up to where you can hold it for minutes at a time.

It is so cool Mom. I do it every break. It makes me stand up taller and it helps my posture. Matthew said my poor posture is what is causing my shoes to wear at that crazy angle. That said, could you order me a new pair of shoes and send them to school? I am going to be a walking fool from now on.

In all seriousness Mom, I really want you and Dad to work on these things. Here they are again: walk, drink water, use salad plates and smaller bowls, and do The Squeeze. They are so easy to do, and you will lose the weight that is putting strain on your heart. Little things over time can make a big difference!

Well Mom, I hope you are doing well. I am doing great. School is going well and I can't wait for my weekly meetings with John and Matthew. My life is really turning around this semester...I can just feel it!

Anyway, just know that I love you and I will come home to visit soon. Just please try the things I told you about. I can tell you more about them when I visit. Please Mom...do it for all of us.

Love you,

Timmy

18

See How You Want to Be

Three weeks have gone by. Timmy's alarm goes off, letting him know officially, the weekend is over.

"Man, it just seems like the weekends fly by," Timmy muttered to himself as he began his morning routine of turning on the TV and listening to the news as he got dressed and ready for school.

"The best thing about Monday is my meeting with John," Timmy thought to himself.

He grabbed his book bag and headed off to the cafeteria to eat breakfast before meeting with John. Timmy has knocked about two minutes off his walk to the cafeteria, and he isn't out of breath like he used to be.

He can't really see a big difference yet, but he definitely feels it. He has lost almost ten pounds in the past three weeks doing the simple things Matthew suggested. If anything, Timmy has really made an effort to "just move" by walking more than he ever has in his entire life.

He loves being outdoors and getting fresh air. Things got even easier about ten days ago as a new pair of shoes arrived in the mail. Wouldn't you know it, walking on flat shoes is much easier than walking on shoes badly worn at an angle.

Timmy arrived at the cafeteria refreshed from his walk, with a light glistening of sweat on his forehead. Standing in line waiting his turn, he pointed his toes straight ahead, squeezed his butt and abs, and pulled his shoulders back tight. He told himself he was going to hold the squeeze until it was his turn.

Almost a minute went by before the line lurched forward. He grabbed a bowl, filled it with frosted flakes and some whole milk, and placed it on the table in the far corner. He went back to the drink bar to get a glass of low-fat milk and a glass of water. He figured that since he is drinking low-fat milk, putting whole milk on his cereal is a good compromise. Besides, it makes him happy.

Timmy finished his breakfast, stood up, did The Squeeze, and headed off on another walk across campus to meet John.

"Morning, Timmy! Just another amazing Monday," said an energetic John.

"Hi, John," replied Timmy in an I-wish-the-weekend-wasn't-over voice.

"You look great, Timmy. I see that you walked over here again this morning, how is that going?"

"It is actually going very well, John. All the stuff Matthew has had me do is really paying off. My posture is getting better. My toes don't point out to the side as much. I am walking a lot and not getting that crazy wear on my shoes where they become slanted, so that is pretty amazing.

"Overall, I feel a lot better. I have lost almost ten pounds. I don't really 'see' it yet, but I definitely feel it."

"I am just so glad to hear that Timmy," replied John. "That leads into what I want to talk to you about today: visualization. Visualization is bar none one of the greatest tools we have in life.

"A wise man once said:

Imagination is more important than knowledge. For knowledge is limited to all we now know and understand, while imagination embraces the entire world, and all there ever will be to know and understand." - Albert Einstein

"You see Timmy, the ability to see what you want, at will, is one of mankind's most prized faculties. Visualization allows your mind to take you anywhere you want to go and be anybody you want to be. If there is something you don't like about yourself or some interaction you had in your life, you can go back to that memory and visualize a different outcome. Similarly, you can skyrocket into the future and see yourself doing great things."

"That sounds pretty cool, John. I often wonder what it would be like to be 180 pounds and not over 300, but I don't really know to visualize that."

"I understand where you are coming from, Timmy. Believe me I do. Most people don't even know what they want, so being able to visualize is very hard for them. The other thing is that most people confuse dreaming with visualizing.

"Timmy, when I ask most people what they want in life, what do you think they say?"

"I don't know," replied Timmy.

"That is exactly right! Most people don't know what they want. So, what do you think they get?"

"Again, I don't know," replied a somewhat confused Timmy.

"That is the problem, Timmy. If people don't know what they want, what do they think life is going to give them? If I don't know what you want for Christmas, and I just get you something random, what are the odds it is going to make you happy?" said John.

"Not very good odds for me," replied Timmy.

"Exactly, that is why you need to visualize what you want out of life. The more that your mind sees an image of it, the more likely it is to come true.

"So Timmy, what is it you would like to visualize? What would you like to see yourself doing, or where would you like to see yourself?"

"You know, John, I really want to see myself at 180 pounds. I want to be active, and I want to be able to do things. The past few years it seems that all of my 'travel' and 'worldly experiences' came from my couch via the TV. I know there is more to life, but it is hard when you get out of breath just from walking across the room."

John looked at Timmy, nodding his head. "I understand completely where you are coming from. I can see you doing the things you want to do. I can see you living life at 180 pounds. The question is, can you?"

"Well, sort of…I guess…I think I can…maybe? I don't know," stammered a clearly uncertain Timmy.

"Well, I have some good news for you. I have yet to have a person that didn't get the concept of visualization or how to do it effectively after I worked with them. I love seeing the look on people's faces when they realize how transformational and important this tool can be to achieving the things they want in life. You will get it too, Timmy. I promise.

"Are you ready to get started?"

"I already visualized us starting," replied Timmy with a sly smirk on his face.

John calmly slapped his hand on Timmy's shoulder and with a smile on his face said, "Very funny, Timmy. I am glad to see your personality coming out, though. I like it and look forward to seeing more of it!

"The first step in visualization is comfort. Before starting, always make sure you're comfortable, whether sitting in a chair, sitting on the floor with your legs crossed, or lying down. There's nothing worse than trying to force yourself to do visualization when you are not comfortable. I like to stretch beforehand so I can relieve tension by loosening up my muscles and joints. I find that this really aids in my ability to relax. Feel free to add cushions, pillows, or blankets as well."

Timmy jokingly asked, "What about my favorite stuffed animal?"

With a straight face, John replies, "If it makes you comfortable, then by all means.

"After you are comfortable, the second thing you need is good posture. If you are sitting up, keep your back straight and not slouched. Keep your head up and your shoulders back. Try to keep this posture comfortable, and for as long as possible. If you are lying down, keep your body straight. It is ok if you have your head on a pillow; just try to keep your chin from digging into your chest. Your head should be resting comfortably on the pillow.

"The third item to focus on is your breathing. Your breathing should be deep, yet very calm. From personal experience, I find using about seventy percent of your capacity of inhalation and exhalation to be a good rule of thumb, especially at the beginning. You don't want to take super long deep breaths, and super long exhalations. The breathing should be natural. The purpose for breathing like this is to enhance relaxation and focus.

"Now that you are comfortable, have good posture, and are breathing efficiently, this is where the rubber meets the proverbial road. This is where you start visualizing what you want. Probably the first things you are going to visualize are images of what you will look like at 180 pounds. You will then visualize yourself doing different activities and going places at this new weight, in your new body."

Timmy looked at John completely serious, "John, I know I want to lose weight, but after that, I don't know what to visualize."

"That is completely understandable, Timmy. The thing is, you can visualize whatever you want. If there is something you want, but you can't visualize it, feel free to look it up online so that you can find pictures of whatever it is, and use those images to help you visualize. The key to doing this is that you don't have to be reasonable in selecting what you want!

"For the sake of this exercise, let's talk about a boat, a house, or a vacation that you want to take."

Timmy perks up, "Ohhhh, I would love a boat."

"That is great. We will use that then. Take a minute and imagine yourself walking down the pier to your boat.

"What does it look like?

"What color is it?

"What does the interior look like?

"What does it smell like?

"Who is there with you?

"Really try and see the boat in all of its detail in your mind.

"If at first you are having problems seeing all of the details, don't sweat it. It's like working out; your muscles aren't used to it at first, but over time you'll get it."

"I can't wait to try this at night when I am lying in bed," said Timmy.

"Funny you say that," said John. "We will discuss it later, but there is something special I like to do every night before bed that falls right in line with this.

"One thing I have found that is very helpful is to call emotion to the images. When you add feelings to images, the feelings are like extra fuel that give your intentions a huge boost, and gets it out into the atmosphere, where it can be realized."

"Hold on, I don't think I get the part about adding emotion to images."

"Thanks for stopping me, Timmy. Let me try to clarify this for you. Have you ever gotten goose bumps or a chill up your spine when you were watching a heroic news story or something amazing on TV? We want to take these emotions and associate them with your desired images. You are creating these things all the time. Maybe cars are your thing; when you see and hear a new Ferrari zip by, you get a chill down your spine. Does that help?"

"Oh, that helps tremendously. The car example really hits home for me. Several months ago, I was driving home and this Lamborghini blew by me. I can't put into words how amazing it sounded. It literally sent a chill down my spine. I went home and watched videos of exotic cars on YouTube for several hours."

"Awesome, Timmy! That is exactly what we want. Doesn't that chill feel good? When you apply an emotion to your visualization, it becomes much more powerful, and much closer to becoming a reality.

"I hope that makes sense."

"It does make sense, but some of it still seems a little hokey to me."

"That is completely understandable, Timmy. Have you ever been around somebody that got a parking ticket, missed a train, or dropped something and they said, 'I knew that was going to happen?' They had visualized something negative happening, and low and behold, it did!

"I am not saying this is easy, Timmy. It is a big mind shift for most people. I know it took me some time to really get it. I couldn't see how positive visualization could work, but it does. After all, it worked for me for years, just with negative things like parking tickets, and other 'bad vibes' that I got, which ended up coming true. I decided to turn things around and use visualization for positive things, and trust me, it works!"

"John, I have learned so much from you and Matthew both, and you are amazing people who are living fulfilling lives. If you guys are doing these things, and I see your results, I would be a fool not to try. I could continue to keep my negative vibes, but I wouldn't get any positive news with that negative attitude."

A large smile crossed John's face, "Matthew said you were a quick learner, and now I see it. You really are wise beyond your years, Timmy. You realize when you start doing these things that your life is going to change in ways you can't even fathom right now. I know that losing weight is first and foremost for you, but you will be amazed what happens when you combine a powerful mind with a healthy body. Watch out, world!

"On that note, let's take a short break as there are two more things I want to talk to you about. How does that sound, Timmy?"

Timmy stood up straight with his chest out and his shoulders back. "Sounds great to me, John. I just need five minutes to get some water and use the restroom."

"Five minutes it is. Ready…break!"

John and Timmy walked out of the office and headed for the water fountain and the restroom.

19

'Snooze' to Success

John and Timmy head back into the office at the same time. Timmy is feeling pretty good about himself as he gives John a playful nudge as they try to go through the door at the same time.

"Was a great break wasn't it, Timmy? It must have been good because now you think you can push me around," said John jokingly.

"Don't mess with me," said Timmy. "I visualized myself being the first one through that door."

John couldn't hold in his laughter any longer and let out a nice chuckle. "Wait until I tell Matthew, I think we have created a monster."

Timmy just sat down with a big grin on his face.

"All righty then...now that we know a bit about visualization, we are going to put it into our daily routine. I am going to teach you the 'Snooze to Success.'

"Some people like to do this drill first thing in the morning when they 'snooze' their alarm clock for five to ten minutes; some people like to do at night before they fall asleep. I think it is best to do it both times.

"At night, you want the last thoughts before you sleep to be positive and inspirational for the four to eight hours where your subconscious mind is very active. Done first thing in the morning, it sets the tone for your day. It doesn't have to be exactly seven minutes, but that is just a good number that I like."

"Ok, but what is it?" enquired Timmy.

"If you haven't read it already, Napoleon Hill, the author of *Think and Grow Rich*, talks about autosuggestion. Autosuggestion is programming your subconscious mind with what you want to have happen.

"You see, Timmy, before you retire into the dream world for four to eight hours where your subconscious mind breaks down your day, you want to put only the best programming in your mind before you nod off to sleep.

"Scientists have been studying people while they sleep for years, and they have discovered this time is crucial for the brain to break down and analyze information it couldn't during the day on a conscious level, in your waking state."

"I'm conscious of what you are saying…but barely," said a smirking Timmy, trying to be funny again.

"The first thing I do is recap the day in my mind; the good, the bad, and everything in between. I am grateful not just for the good things that happened, but for the bad as well. You have to change your mindset to look at 'bad things' as merely challenges or opportunities to overcome to make you a stronger person."

Timmy squinted at John and shot him a serious look. "Believe it or not, this makes sense to me. The mind is powerful. If Matthew had told me before my mom's heart attack about the simple ways to lose weight, I wouldn't have been in the right mindset to hear it, or want his help. I now believe that I can change my life by doing things that have a positive effect on my mind."

"Great attitude to have, Timmy! Your attitude is a big reason why you are seeing results with your weight loss. Just wait, you will start seeing positive things show up in other areas of your life as well."

"I know. I can't wait. It is just nice to wake up and look forward to the day."

"Lastly, I encourage you to partake in a short exercise. What I want you to do is create what is called 'The Day Script.' What you are going to do is write a short paragraph or two of what you would like to see happen tomorrow. Here are some questions to ask yourself:

- Who is involved?
- Where are you going?

- What's the weather like?
- Who's going to call you?
- Whose life are you going to impact?"

"These are all questions you can ask yourself in those last remaining minutes before bed. It will make a difference. I encourage you to adopt this life changing habit as it is an amazing technique for bringing more peace, control, and positive outcomes into your life.

"When you wake up in the morning, I suggest hitting the snooze button one time, and taking that time to visualize how you want your day to turn out. You can answer those same questions as above, or you can visualize your success at a big meeting or presentation you might have that day.

"If you prime your subconscious mind before you sleep and prime your conscious mind before your day starts, you can't help but start and end your day on a positive note! How does that sound, Timmy?"

"I have to be honest with you. I have heard about this stuff before, and I was skeptical. The thing is, I might be skeptical, but it just dawned on me that the only people I hear of doing this are successful people! So I guess I would be a fool not to do what works for them."

"Great point, Timmy. I used to be the same way, but finally figured it was worth trying for a month. It isn't something that will change you after only one time, but if you commit to it and make it a habit, you will notice positive changes in your life!"

Nodding in agreement, Timmy said, "I hear you John. I am going to start tonight. I am going to recap my day and think about what I want to accomplish tomorrow. I will give my subconscious some good stuff to feast on. When I wake up in the morning, I will set the tone for my day. I mean, really. How hard is this to do? It is seven minutes before you fall asleep and seven minutes when you wake up.

"I have to be honest with you, John; I was expecting some sort of rocket science or crazy hard work from you and Matthew, but in reality, both of you have me doing little things that make a big difference. It isn't overwhelming at all. Heck, all you have to do is make these little changes over time, and you will see big results. I like it!"

With a big smile on his face, John put his arm around Timmy and said, "I am so excited to be working with you. Matthew is right; I also see big things in your future. Now let's take another quick break as I have one more thing to discuss with you today.

"On a side note, you try and bump me again and see what happens there, buddy. Have a good break, and I will see you in five."

Just as John moved his arm from around Timmy, Timmy gave him a little bump and laughed as he skirted out the door and down the hall.

"Oh Timmy..." exclaimed John with a big smile on his face.

20

Affirmation Station

Timmy *returns from the break, wiping drops of water that dribbled down his chin from the water fountain.*

"All right. I know you have a class coming up in a little while, but we have time to discuss one more little trick that I like to use."

Bleep…bleep…bleep…went John's cell phone sitting on the desk.

"Aren't you going to answer that?" asked Timmy quizzically.

"Nope. Because that isn't a phone call."

"Uhh…ok. Whatever," muttered Timmy rolling his eyes as if his mentor was crazy.

"Don't 'whatever' me," said John. "Read what it says."

John handed the phone to Timmy, who read the screen, "I am amazing and made in God's likeness."

"What is this?" asked Timmy.

"It is what I like to call 'affirmation station.' Go ahead and get out your cell phone."

"Ok. This is a first; a teacher wants me to *take out* my cell phone instead of putting it away or turning it off," said Timmy with a sarcastic tone to his voice.

"What we are going to do is set alarms to go off throughout the day that will give your mind powerful, positive impressions multiple times per day. You can set them to be every hour, or every couple of hours; it is up to you."

"I'm not sure I get it yet," said an inquisitive Timmy.

"What we want to do is make a list of at least ten affirmations that we want to tell ourselves throughout the day. These affirmations can be anything positive you want to tell yourself or things you want to work on."

Nodding his head in agreement, Timmy asked, "Do they have to be religious? I saw that in your affirmation you mentioned God. Do I have to do that?"

"That is a great question. No, it doesn't have to be religious. For me, I believe in having and working on my spiritual side. Your affirmations are up to you. I know people that put things about health, procrastination, or being successful, while others put bible verses or religious quotes. Some even put their affirmations in Hebrew or another language.

"You want to put affirmations, or positive thoughts, into your mind with whatever you are working on at the time. For you, I can see you putting affirmations like 'I am losing weight,' 'I am athletic,' 'I am confident,' and 'People are drawn to me.' Does that help it to make more sense?"

"That is really cool!" said a perked up Timmy. "So I need to make a list of all the things I want to work on, then set alarms to go off throughout the day with the title of each alarm being whatever my affirmation is. Is it that easy?"

"You nailed it! And yes, it is that easy," said John with a big smile on his face.

"You can write anything you wish, like…

'I no longer hold onto the past.'
'I'm made in the image and the likeness of God.'
'Money comes to me easily.'
'Everything I touch turns to gold.'
'My relationships are in complete harmony.'
'I am amazing and people are drawn to me.'
'I am a success!'

"I think you get the point. The affirmations can be anything. The cool thing about this is that it is so simple to do, doesn't take much time, and it really works!"

"I totally see how easy it is," said Timmy. "But are you sure it really works?"

"I understand why you are skeptical, but the reason it works so well is because I know you have had those days where your 'negative' mind has taken over and is starting to get you down. Maybe you stumbled on your diet and ate a whole pizza, or procrastinated on a homework assignment, or maybe your mind was telling you that you will always be overweight.

"Just then, your phone goes off, which interrupts that negative voice in your head. You pick up your phone to see a positive affirmation that boosts your confidence and kicks your positive mental attitude back into gear."

"I see," said Timmy. "So true. The negative voice can get quite powerful sometimes."

"Yes it can. But when you have positive affirmations going off every hour, or multiple times per day, it really helps keep you in a positive frame of mind. Often times, we know how good we are, but we let that 'other' voice start talking to us. These affirmations remind us of how good we really are and keep us on track.

"I wouldn't be telling you this if it didn't work and if I didn't do it myself. You saw one alarm go off." As John opens the alarm application on his phone, "and here is the list of the other alarms that I have set."

"Wow, pretty cool," said Timmy. "I really like it when people actually practice what they preach."

"I wouldn't have it any other way," said John. "One thing I will tell you is that when your phone is on vibrate, make sure the alarm is set to vibrate as well. I got a surprise before when my phone was vibrating but the alarm was still set to make a sound. Just something to be aware of so your alarm doesn't make noise during a meeting, test, or other inopportune time."

"I am definitely going to do this, John. That said, I need to start walking so I can make my first class today."

"Good to see that you are watching the clock and are sticking with your walking to class commitment. I am really proud of you, Timmy. You have come a long way in just a few short weeks. Wait until you see the difference over the next few months and even years as you keep making small positive changes to your life."

"Thanks, John! I am really enjoying our meetings and the ones with Matthew as well." Timmy stood up straight and held it for a few seconds. "I am off to class!" And with that, he headed out the door.

"Keep up the great work, Timmy!" shouted John as Timmy rounded the corner down the hall.

Letter to Mom #3

Tuesday, September 28

Dear Mom,

How are you doing? I need you to do me a quick favor. I need for you to stand up and do The Squeeze while you read this. Stop rolling your eyes, Mom, and do it for me. I have a lot of things I want to share with you.

Remember those simple things I told you to do from my last letter…walk, water, portion size, and the stretchercise? Well, they work! Guess how much weight I have lost? Almost 10 pounds…of pure body fat! I should be less than 300 pounds here soon! I know what you are thinking, that it is going to come back, but trust me mom, it won't. I made a lifestyle change, not a short-term change.

That said, I have learned so much lately, I almost don't know where to start. I guess going back a few weeks and starting there makes the most sense.

Since Matthew was working with me on the physical side of things, John started teaching me about the super important mental side of things. I had no idea the mind was so powerful.

John taught me how to use my mind to visualize what I want to accomplish in life. You can do this easily because you are laying down quite a bit. The important thing is to be calm, and take "70 percent breaths." Not too deep on the way in and not all the way out.

When you get into this calm state, think about how you want things to be. Think about yourself walking on the beach with Dad and being healthy again. Think of being there for Jessica's, Jason's, and my children. You still have decades of life to live; you just have to visualize the way you want it to be.

I know making time to visualize can be tough, that is why John taught me this amazing tool called "the last 7 minutes." Basically, you are just visualizing for the 7 minutes before you fall asleep. I take it to the next level by visualizing for 7 minutes when I wake up during my snooze in the morning, too.

At night, I visualize how my day was, and I look at the opportunity hidden within all of my daily challenges. This allows me to see obstacles, not as obstacles, but as opportunities, which I make into positive experiences. It is also very important to put positive thoughts into the mind before you sleep, because the subconscious mind is very active at night.

Then, first thing in the morning when my alarm goes off, I hit the snooze button and lie there for 7 minutes, visualizing how good my day is going to be. I see my day in my mind before it happens.

It is really funny Mom, you know how you would always say, and "I just knew that was going to happen…" whenever you hit a red light or it rained or something else "bad" happened? I find the same thing happening to me; it is just with good stuff though! I was skeptical at first, but working on my mind has helped me so much.

You have to see it in your mind before it can become real. You can be active and at a healthy weight again, you just have to start seeing it for yourself. I see you being that person again, Mom; I just hope you can too.

I know those things can take a bit of time, but the last thing John showed me takes no time at all. He calls it "affirmation station." So get out your cell phone. Go ahead, I know it isn't very far from reach because it never is. Ha-ha…just kidding with you, Mom.

Anyway, take your phone and I want you to set 4-5 alarms to go off throughout the day. For each alarm that goes off, I want you to write an affirmation. You could put stuff like:

I am healthy and losing weight.
I will be there for my grandchildren.
I am an amazing mother.
God is by my side.
Money comes to me easily.

Write down whatever you want to motivate you. When your phone goes off during the day, you will look down, see those things, and it will automatically get or keep you in a positive state of mind.

Just trust me on this, Mom! Do the visualization before you fall asleep and when you wake up, and do the affirmation station for 3 weeks in a row. You will not be disappointed!

It is still a few weeks away, but I think Jason is going to try and come visit me for the homecoming weekend. I'm not a big fan of crowds and walking around, but I have to say it is getting a lot easier for me. So I am sort of looking forward to the big game.

Anyway, tell Dad and Jessica I'm doing great and I miss them. I will probably come home around Thanksgiving, maybe sooner. We'll see.

Take care of yourself, Mom! I look forward to seeing a difference when I see you again. I am sure you will be able to see a difference with me.

I love you Mom…

Little Timmy (ha ha…I'm getting there!)

22

Motivation Strikes

BRAAAK...BRAAAK...BRAAAK...broke the early morning silence as the rather annoying clock radio went off. Like a guided missile, Timmy's left arm sprang from the covers, flew wildly out to the side behind him, and his index finger landed dead on the snooze button.

"Ah, silence," Timmy thought to himself. He lay there motionless for about two minutes before starting his "7 minutes to success" ritual, which had become part of his morning snooze routine like John had suggested.

Timmy was especially excited about Friday because his brother Jason was coming in town for the Homecoming football game.

He lay there envisioning how perfect the weekend was going to be. From showing Jason around the school, to watching the football game together on Saturday, it was going to be one amazing weekend.

Timmy was proud of himself. Over the past 6 weeks he had lost about 15 pounds just by walking, drinking water, and watching his portion control. He had noticed a big difference in his energy levels and self-confidence, but he hadn't seen a big difference in the mirror yet. He was closing in on 305 pounds on the scale, but he knew in just a few more weeks he would be less than 300 pounds.

BRAAAK…BRAAAK…BRAAAK…went the alarm again. It was time to get up and start his day.

As Timmy finished getting dressed, he picked up his shoes and inspected the soles. "Not bad," he thought to himself.

He had been walking a lot the past six weeks, and his shoes were wearing better than they had in years. There was still some uneven wear, but nothing like it was. "Matthew and his stretchercise, 'The Squeeze,' have really helped me correct my posture," Timmy thought out loud as he sat on the corner of his bed to put his shoes on.

All Timmy could think about on his walk to the cafeteria was that Jason was on his way into town. He couldn't wait to show him around campus, and he wanted to see if Jason would notice the new Timmy.

Jason was a few years older and still lived at home because it was cheaper and he wasn't around much anyway because of work. He was a workhorse for a large tree farm and landscaping company where he worked long hours in what could be described as a pretty physical job. Jason always liked getting his hands dirty and knew that a life behind a desk wasn't for him.

He wasn't as heavy as Timmy, but definitely overweight. Thinking back to his talks with Matthew, Timmy knew his brother was "moving," but he also knew Jason ate whatever he wanted and liked his alcohol. One thing Jason liked to do was jog on the treadmill they had at work, but even with the extra jogging he still couldn't lose weight.

Timmy looked forward to Jason's arrival and hoped Jason would not only notice a difference in his weight, but also want to make some life changes for himself. Timmy wanted his entire family to experience his new outlook on life.

Timmy received two tickets to the homecoming football game from John and Matthew. He was excited but also apprehensive about going. Even though he was feeling great, losing weight, and gaining confidence, he was still nervous and self-conscious when around large groups of people.

Timmy still believed that people were staring at him and making comments about his weight. He was afraid of what they may be thinking about him. Taming that voice in his head was going to take time, but the visualization tools were definitely helping. He found stopping the stream of negative thoughts and replacing them with positive ones was a key task to success.

"Please take one and pass it along," said the teacher, interrupting Timmy's daydream.

Timmy passed the papers along. "Lunchtime can't come soon enough," he thought to himself, not because he was hungry, but because Jason should be meeting him for lunch.

He sat through two classes but was so anxious to see his brother; nothing the teachers said penetrated his mind. He was too busy thinking about his brother and visualizing the next two days in his mind.

After what seemed like an eternity, the dull alarm that signified class was over finally went off. "This weekend is going to be amazing," is all he could think to himself.

A huge smile crossed Timmy's face as he grabbed his notebook, stood up, and headed to go meet Jason.

Timmy hustled his way towards the cafeteria that was near one of the smaller, lesser-known lots for guest parking. As he got closer, he was scanning the lot for Jason's pickup truck.

"Ah, there it is," he muttered to himself with a sense of excitement. He could see Jason's pickup truck across the parking lot. No way to miss the slightly lifted work truck with the big CB whip-antenna on top. Even with cell phones, the landscaping company still used CB radio as a means to communicate.

Timmy was excited and began to walk even faster.

WHAM! Out of nowhere Timmy felt a vice like grip on his right arm, just below his shoulder.

"Where you going, speed walker?"

Timmy whipped around to the right shaking free of the grip.

"Holy crap!"

Upon seeing a friendly face, the tension melted away.

Hitting his brother playfully in the chest, "Gosh-darn-it Jason, you scared the crap out of me!"

"Ha-ha. Let me look at you. Are you feeling ok? Your face looks thinner. Are you sick or fighting off a cold?"

A big smile crossed Timmy's face. Even though he couldn't see the changes by looking in the mirror every day, it was obvious that Jason noticed a difference, as they hadn't seen each other since the weekend Mom had the heart attack.

"What do you mean?"

"Come on. You had to have lost some weight. Your face looks thinner, less round. Have you been sick or something?"

"No, I haven't been sick at all," said Timmy, somewhat offended. "I have been changing my habits so that I can lose weight."

"Really? Mom said you wrote her some letter and that you were going to try and lose weight. Well, good luck. Don't get down on yourself when the weight comes back. I have a job where I am pretty active and I can't lose any weight, so I have just come to accept that this is the way our family is."

"That isn't true, Jason. We don't have to be this way. Let's get something to eat and we can talk about it."

"Sounds good because I am starving after the drive."

Jason threw his arm across Timmy's shoulder as they turned around and started walking towards the cafeteria.

As they entered, Timmy told Jason to get his food and to meet him at the table in the far corner.

Jason took a minute to survey the cafeteria and look at all of the options he had for lunch. After all, he was starving.

Timmy grabbed one of the smaller salad plates like he had been doing for six weeks, went through the main line, grabbed a big glass of water, and headed to the corner table.

A minute later, Jason walked over and set down a large glass of soda with a heaping plate of food.

"I will be right back. Saw some good eats in the a-la-carte line."

Jason returned shortly with two small plates containing a slice of pizza and some onion rings.

"What's up with the baby plate, Timmy? You are sick aren't you? Eat up, boy."

"Jason, that is what I am talking about. Look at all the food you have in front of you."

"I'm starving. What don't you get?"

"I get that you are hungry, but 3 plates of food and a big glass of soda is 'why' we can't lose weight."

"Listen Tim, I am older than you and I know that we aren't ever going to be a skinny family. I work hard, burn a lot of calories, even jog a couple days a week, and I can't lose weight. That is just the way we are."

Shaking his head and looking at Jason with eyes that say, "You just don't get it," Timmy wished that he could help Jason see what he has seen.

"Jason, I don't know much about nutrition or anything like that yet. But I have learned a few key points that are easy to do, and they have helped me tremendously," he says as he dips one of the chicken fingers into honey mustard sauce.

"I have lost over fifteen pounds in the past several weeks. You noticed it yourself. You thought I was sick or had been sick.

"I haven't been sick at all; in fact, I have been healthier than ever. I walk everywhere I go, I drink water, and I eat my meals on smaller plates. It isn't rocket science, but I can't argue with the results."

Timmy leaned to the side, grabbed his jeans by his knee, picked his foot up, and plopped it onto the table. "Look at the soles of my shoes. I have been working on my posture so that I don't have the 'sloped shoes' you used to make fun of me for."

"Come on Timmy, get your feet off the table. I am trying to eat here," said Jason as he stuffed the slice of pizza into his mouth. "I'm happy for you, Timmy. I really am. But can we just enjoy our meal and have fun this weekend? I don't want to talk about dieting or losing weight or whatever. I just want to watch some football and hang out with you."

"Fair enough. Just know that I am going to do this, and at some point, I hope that you will want to make some changes too. It is only because I care about you, and the rest of the family."

"So, how are they looking for the big homecoming game tomorrow?" asked Jason in a not-so-subtle way of changing the subject.

"They are looking pretty good from what I hear. I haven't been to any games yet this year because I usually try to avoid crowds."

"And the walking and stairs," quipped Jason.

"Very funny. Those don't bother me anymore. In fact, I am looking forward to walking around tomorrow. It is going to be a fun day!"

"Amen to that," replied Jason, dunking his onion ring into a pile of ranch dressing.

Timmy was disappointed that Jason wasn't very interested in making changes. He was a little surprised that his own achievements weren't enough to make Jason at least a little excited. He understood change was hard and it was easier for most people to keep the status quo than look in the mirror and see what could be done better.

"Oh well," thought Timmy. "I'm not giving up. I will just have to show him what is possible."

Saturday finally arrived. Jason and Timmy found their way into the massive parking lot and found a nice place to park where they should be able to exit quickly after the game. It wasn't the closest spot to the stadium, but Timmy had Jason convinced that walking didn't bother him anymore.

It was a beautiful fall day and the sun was out. It was the kind of day where you could easily be comfortable in jeans and a t-shirt as long as you were in the sun, but once the sun began to set you knew a warm jacket had better be close.

Timmy and Jason were hanging by the pickup listening to music. Jason was drinking his customary beer, and Timmy was drinking a sugar-free Red Bull, looking for an energy kick.

"Hey Timmy, look at 'Mr. Cool Guy' over there."

Timmy turned and looked where Jason was pointing.

"Dude thinks he is so cool just because he looks like Superman in his jeans and t-shirt. He was just born lucky. Guys like that make me sick."

Jason took another big swig of his beer and turned to Timmy, but he was gone.

"Hey Matthew!" shouted Timmy as he walked towards him.

Matthew turned around. "Hey Timmy, how's it going?"

"It's going well, I guess."

"You guess? What could be wrong? It is a beautiful day for some homecoming football!"

"I know, it's just my brother…"

"That's right; your brother is in town, isn't he?"

"Yeah, that's right."

"Is he here? I want to meet him."

"I don't know, Matthew; he isn't totally supportive of my losing weight and all. He thinks it will just come right back. He is sort of a downer about it. And, uhhh…"

"What is it, Timmy?"

"Well, he saw you before I did. And he said some…"

"Stop right there Timmy. You don't have to say anything. I completely understand. It is a natural defense mechanism for people. I would still like to meet him if you are ok with it."

"Yeah, I would like for you to meet him. Maybe if he meets you he will change his attitude a little bit."

"Sure thing. Let me refresh my drink and we can go meet him."

"Wait a second, you're having a drink?"

"You bet, Timmy! I am human like everybody else. I enjoy having a few drinks on occasion. I don't drink all the time, and I don't drink to excess, but I love my vodka soda with lemon!" A big smile crossed Matthew's face. "Everything in moderation!"

Timmy smiled and walked with Matthew towards Jason's truck.

"Hey Jason, I want you to meet Matthew. He is the guy that is helping me out with all of the health and fitness stuff. He is a good friend of John, who is my counselor. Between the two of them, they are helping me transform my life. Not to mention that they got us the tickets to the game!"

"Hey, uh, nice to meet you," said Jason with his head down a little bit and his eyes staying low.

"It is a pleasure to meet you, Jason. Timmy has had nothing but great things to say about you. How are things with the tree and landscaping business?"

Somewhat taken back, "Oh, uh, um, things are fine. Thanks for asking."

"The first thing he noticed when he saw me was that my face looked thinner. Right Jason?" Timmy said proudly.

"Yeah, that's right. I thought he had been sick or something."

"Hey Timmy, why don't you grab money from my wallet and buy a program from the guy over there?" Jason asked.

"Sure thing," said Timmy as he grabbed a five-dollar bill from the console of the pickup.

"Can I talk to you for a second, Matthew?" Jason said.

"Sure thing, what is it, Jason?"

"I really appreciate what you are doing with Timmy, I just don't want him to get hurt when whatever diet you have him on stops working and he puts all his weight back on."

"I completely understand where you are coming from, and nobody wants to see a loved one have their hopes dashed. The thing is, I don't have Timmy on any diet or program. It is about making small changes that yield big returns and once he makes them part of his lifestyle, he will have them for the rest of his life. There is no 'quick fix' to anything he is doing. In fact, it is quite the contrary."

"I have to admit, I was surprised when I saw him. Not only was he walking pretty fast, but also I could see that he had lost weight in his face. It is just that he is so overweight, and our whole family is that way. Mom and Dad have tried diets, but they never worked. That is just the way we are. We aren't lucky like you, Matthew."

"I appreciate your noticing Timmy's achievement. The thing is, I believe that he is going to do it. It is just a matter of changing habits. Sure, some people might have better genetics for being thin than others, just like some people are smarter than others. But really, it all comes down to habits.

"I might not be as smart as somebody else, so what does that mean? It means I have to study more. Just as your family might not be as naturally lean as another family means you just have to work at it a bit more. That's all.

"Trust me, I know it is hard. I had a roommate in college who as a freshman was taking classes with juniors and seniors. And get this...he was always playing video games! I was fighting my way to get C's in freshman classes, and he was getting A's in advanced classes...and he wasn't even studying! Trust me, I hated it. But just because he was playing video games and not studying, didn't mean I could do the same thing. Does that make sense?

"Timmy is going to get there. All I ask is that you watch him change as a person and support him along the way. I know it isn't going to be easy, but he is doing great so far. If he keeps it up, he will be less than 300 pounds here soon, and if he changes nothing else, he will be less than 200 pounds in another two years. Not bad results for some simple lifestyle changes with no diets or programs involved."

"I hear what you are saying," said Jason, taking another big drink of his beer. "I will do all I can to support him. Heck, you look like you obviously know what you are talking about, so if it works for Timmy, I might just give it a shot."

"That is all I can ask of you. That said, I really believe Timmy is going to be able to help a lot of people. I know he is your younger brother, but don't be afraid to learn from him."

"Here you go, Jason." Timmy walked up and handed Jason the program for the game. "What are you guys talking about?"

"Jason was just telling me how much of an improvement he had noticed and that he was proud of you." Matthew explained.

Timmy couldn't help but beam and stand taller. It was just the thing he needed to put a little extra spring in his step.

Jason just looked at Matthew, giving him a subtle nod to say thanks.

"You guys enjoy the game. I have to go meet some people as they have my ticket. Jason, it was great to finally meet you. Have a great day, guys!"

"Thanks again, Matthew," said Timmy.

Jason stuck out his hand to shake Matthew's hand. "Thanks. I will think about what you said."

"You about ready to head into the game?" Timmy asked Jason. "I want to get to our seats and soak in everything homecoming has to offer."

"Fine by me. Let me finish this beer and we can go in."

About thirty minutes later they were in the stadium, walking down a long flight of stairs towards their seats.

"Let me see your ticket," asked Jason. "Are our seats really that close to the field?"

"Yes, they are," said an enthusiastic Timmy.

They made their way down the steps to their seats, which were impressive. They were dead even with the goal line only about 20 rows up.

"I am going to go grab a beer, you want anything?" asked Jason.

"Nah, I'm all right. Thanks though."

Jason turned and left for the concession stands.

Timmy was just standing there, taking in all of the activity on this beautiful fall day. His eyes were fluttering around the stadium. It was so much different than playing Madden on his Sony PlayStation. The energy flowing through the stadium was so real.

Then he froze. It was as if Timmy had seen a ghost. He stood there in a trance looking down at the field. Could it really be?

There she was, like an angel on the sidelines. Natalie Williams.

Natalie was one of the cheerleaders. She had a smile that would light up a room and cut through even the toughest frown. She had lightly tanned skin that just seemed to glow right along with her personality and positive energy. Her long brown hair made her blue eyes pop like you wouldn't believe.

Her body was firm, yet feminine and curvaceous. She was gorgeous. She was the girl next door. She was the girl every guy on campus dreamed about, and every girl dreamed of becoming.

Timmy stood there as if time stood still. He was lost in the idea of Natalie. For a moment in time, he felt like a 190-pound chiseled athlete. He felt light on his feet, and everything in the world was right.

His stomach had this warm sensation inside. He veins felt warm as this energy and passion ran through his body. Timmy was just enjoying the feeling that had washed over him.

Then it happened. Natalie looked up right at Timmy. His gaze was immediately focused on those captivating blue eyes. He was drawn in like a fly to a Venus-fly-trap. How could he possibly resist something so sweet and something that had every nerve ending in his body on fire?

He couldn't.

He was trapped in her eyes. Without having any real control over his body, he did what felt natural. Holding his gaze with her, he picked up his right arm and waved. Timmy felt strong and confident waving his hand at her. After all, in this moment, he was the only man in the world that mattered.

On the outside though, this wasn't the kind of wave you see between friends or one made with confidence. No, this wave was the kind you see in movies. Those movies where the dorky kid tries to steal the girl from the quarterback jock.

On the inside it felt so right, so strong, and so powerful. On the outside, it looked so awkward, so forced, so unnatural.

But it didn't matter. She saw him.

Her smile widened as if she was trying to light up the stadium. She raised her arm and waved like pretty cheerleaders have done thousands of times before, but there was something special about this wave. There was something extra in it. It was as if this wave was meant for him.

The energy running through his body was unlike anything he had ever felt before. For the shy, chubby kid, this was a huge leap forward. Timmy felt amazing. He even started to sway back and forth as he still kept waving with a big smile on his face.

As he was swaying, something caught the corner of his eye. Turning slightly, he looked over his right shoulder. What he saw would change him forever. It was like a switch had been thrown. All of the warm energy running through his body ceased in an instant. The warmth in his stomach was replaced by a feeling similar to a sucker-punch from Mike Tyson.

Standing above Timmy off to the right, was in fact "Mr. Right." Or at least that is what he looked like to Timmy. He was tall, lean, and athletic, but worst of all, he had a big smile on his face, and he too was waving at Natalie.

Only about five seconds had passed since his gaze first met Natalie's, but it seemed like an eternity. His head swiveled back towards Natalie, only to see her blow a kiss towards him, which he painfully knew was actually Mr. Right's direction.

He heard a muffled voice that brought him back to reality.

"Hey Timmy, will you grab this for me?"

It was Jason coming back from the concession stand.

"I know you said you didn't want anything, but I grabbed you two hot dogs and a soda. I grabbed two beers and a couple of hot dogs myself so I didn't have to wait in line again."

Timmy looked at Jason with eyes that were empty. He grabbed one of the large beers and drank it faster than a person rescued in the desert drinks water.

He crushed the plastic cup and threw it to the ground. He picked up the other beer and chugged half of it, before pausing to eat an entire hot dog in one bite.

Jason stood there in disbelief.

"Are you ok? What happened? I wasn't gone that long."

Timmy's eyes communicated all that Jason needed to know at the moment.

"All righty then. I'm going to go get more beer, you want anything else?"

Timmy continued to stare off into space.

The rest of the day became nothing more than just a blur. After a few more beers and hot dogs, Jason finally had to throw in the towel and get Timmy home.

They left before halftime. On their way out of the stadium, Jason heard a familiar voice.

"Jason…Timmy, where are you guys going?"

Jason turned to see Matthew walking towards them.

"What happened?"

"I have no idea. He was having a great time when we got to the seats. I left to go hit the concession stands and when I came back it was like he was a different person. He just started chugging the beer and eating hot dogs," Jason explained as Timmy continued walking towards the truck.

"Hmmm. Well, I will talk with him next week. That just doesn't sound like him."

"I know. I really have no idea what happened during that time when I went to get food. I am going to take him home. Will you do me a favor, Matthew?"

"Sure, what is it?"

"Will you help my little brother? I know he really looks up to you. With you, he has a shot at being the first person in our family to not go through life overweight. He is young and has a shot at turning it all around. I really want him to be happy."

A comforting smile crossed Matthew's face. "You got it, Jason. I am and will do everything I can to help him. Get that kid some rest and I will discuss this with him next week."

"Thank you so much, Matthew. I am so fortunate that he met people like you and John that truly care about him. Most people outside of the family just write us off as being overweight and lazy, and it just isn't the case."

"I understand, Jason. Society as a whole likes to make snap judgments about people, and more often than not, they are wrong."

"You don't ever make judgments about people, do you Jason?" asked Matthew with an inquisitive look on his face.

Jason saw the look on his face and thought back to what he had said earlier about the "random" guy that turned out to be Matthew.

"I…I try not to, but it happens sometimes," said Jason sheepishly.

"It's ok. We are all human. All we can do is apologize and catch ourselves when we slip, and work on making ourselves better people."

"That is very true. Thanks again for the tickets and everything else. It was a pleasure to meet you, and I look forward to watching Timmy evolve as a person."

"You're welcome, Jason. Have a good afternoon, and I am sure we will meet again at some point."

"For sure," replied Jason as he turned away and headed for the truck.

Timmy woke up late Sunday morning with a hangover. It took him a few minutes to get his bearings and figure out where he was, what time it was, and how he got there.

After a few minutes and a stop by the bathroom to throw some water on his face, he ventured out to the living room to see if Jason was still there. The blankets were folded up on the couch and there were two empty pizza boxes from what appeared to be dinner.

He couldn't remember much about the rest of the day after the "Natalie incident," but his dry mouth and banging headache did suggest he needed some water.

As Timmy got close to the refrigerator he saw a note taped to the door:

T,

I had a great time visiting you this weekend. I had to get back this afternoon to get a few things done, and I didn't want to wake you.

Don't worry about yesterday. I don't know what happened; you can tell me later if you want. Something obviously bothered you.

That said...things are really looking up for you, kid! You are doing great losing weight, and I can already see the positive changes you are making. Sorry for what I said about Matthew yesterday. I didn't know who he was when I said it, but that shouldn't matter. I did to him what people do to us. Matthew is a great guy and I am really glad you have him in your life.

Keep up the great work. I am so proud of you. I will tell the family you are doing great as well.

Love you...

J

A tear began to work its way out of the corner of Timmy's eye and fall gently to his cheek. He wasn't sure if it was because of the incident with Natalie, the fact that his brother wrote a note that said he supported and loved him, or some combination of the two. His emotions were being pulled in so many directions and he really needed to clear his head.

Before Timmy could make sense of all the feelings he was experiencing, he looked back at the empty pizza boxes. He couldn't remember if he even ate pizza or not. There was only one way to find out.

He made his way to the bathroom and stepped on the scale. When he looked down he was crushed.

Somehow he had gained 7 pounds since he last weighed himself a few days ago. Timmy knew it had to have been the beer, hot dogs, and obviously the pizza. What had he done? Weeks of work down the drain, erased in one drunken blur. What was he trying to do to himself? Guilt and regret swept over his body like high tide overtaking a sand bar. He felt like such a loser. Why was life so unfair?

He stepped off the scale and stood in front of the mirror. Unable to control his emotions any longer, a wave of tears came streaming down his face. This was not the kind of life he wanted. This is not what he imagined it would be like. He stood in front of the mirror for what seemed like an eternity. He wasn't looking at himself in a narcissistic sort of way; it was way more serious than that. He stared at himself like a man looking deep into his own soul to see what he was really made of.

It was at that moment, standing in front of the mirror that a new fire burned inside of Timmy, a fire inside that had never burned before. Something clicked. From this day forward he vowed that he was no longer going to be the 300-pound outcast, insecure, scared of people, and avoiding relationships. He loved the feeling he felt when he thought Natalie was flirting with him. It set his soul ablaze, and he wanted to experience it again and again. But he knew that girls didn't find 300-plus pound guys like him attractive, especially when he didn't even like himself.

The reality was sinking in that Timmy was almost 20 years old and he had never gone on a date, much less held hands or kissed a woman. He knew that if he didn't lose weight, it would be very hard to find a woman that would be attracted to him. But more important than that, he knew that his weight was an anchor, dragging his self-confidence down and holding him back in all areas of his life. He knew what he had to do. He was going to change. If he didn't care about or love himself, why would anybody else?

Timmy closed his eyes and let his imagination run wild. He saw himself passionate, self-confident, powerful, kind, funny, and, of course, lean. More importantly, he saw himself happy. He knew that once he felt that way about himself, he would have no problem finding others that would feel that way about him too.

He knew he would be able to get the girl. Maybe not Natalie Williams, but he would find his own "Natalie" that would stir up those same feelings he felt at the football game. He desperately wanted to love and be loved. He wanted that warm feeling to pulse through his veins like electricity when he thought of, looked at, or touched that special someone.

Nothing was going to stop him. The fear of being alone for the rest of his life bore a hole right through him. No way was he going to spend his life alone, bankrupt of self-confidence, and with nothing but the negative thoughts in his head.

Until the past few weeks, the direction he had been heading in life wasn't going to take him to that happy place. Instead, he was headed to a place full of bitterness, excuses, and regrets. He had lived his whole life not knowing there was an alternative, but between his encounter with Natalie and seeing so many people loving life at the football game, it opened his eyes.

He vowed then and there that he would not be one of those angry and bitter people that thought the world was out to get him. He committed himself to gaining self-confidence and losing weight. Those were the only two things holding him back from a world of opportunity.

Timmy turned away from the mirror. In those few short minutes, he became a man on a mission. He was transformed. No longer was he a helpless victim with no control over his life. He understood half the battle was his own thinking, and he didn't have to wait until he reached a perfect weight to start changing his mindset and projecting self-confidence.

He realized that as painful as it was, his encounter with Natalie just might have saved him. In those few brief minutes on a Saturday afternoon, she showed him what was possible in life--happiness beyond anything he had ever known. Not the fleeting happiness that came and went with cheeseburgers and video games, but true happiness that can only come from within, happiness that comes only from loving and accepting yourself.

He knew Natalie couldn't give that feeling of happiness to him. Until he could accept the reality of where he was headed and make the necessary changes so he could be happy with himself first, he knew that true happiness would remain out of reach.

Armed with his newfound freedom and outlook on life, Timmy decided to take the rest of the day to himself. He was going to clean up his place, get some homework done, write a letter to Mom, and get ready for the week. Not to mention he wanted to go on a long walk to enjoy the fresh air and clear the thoughts in his head. After all, he knew he had a lot of work in front of him. He was ready.

Before cleaning up the place, he got out his computer and shot Matthew a quick email:

Matthew,
I am ready to take things to the next level. I can't wait for our meeting this week.
See you soon,
Timmy

He then began to tidy up the place, tossing out the pizza boxes and clearing his mind. Not five minutes later, he heard a ding on his computer. It was an email from Matthew.

Timmy,
I'm glad to hear that. I don't know if you remember, but I ran into you and Jason as you were leaving the game. Don't worry about whatever happened, we can discuss it when we meet. Just put it behind you, live in the present, and look to the future.
"Often times it is our greatest setback that is the best time for a positive advancement."

Looking forward to our meeting!

Matthew

Timmy smiled. He really was lucky to have Matthew in his life. Knowing that he had a "superhero" in his corner really helped his self-confidence.

He was starting to feel good again. Not only were his headache and the accompanying hangover fading away, but for the first time in a long time, he was excited for tomorrow. Matthew was right; whatever happened in the past did not have to determine how he lived his future. He could learn from all his mistakes and poor choices instead of repeating them. It was up to him.

The possibility of living life with confidence, vitality, and fearlessness were all Timmy could think about that day. In addition to actually being able to visualize himself at a normal weight of 180 pounds, he began to visualize what he wanted his life to look like. He thought of the contributions to society he could make, he thought of the people he could help, he thought of the special people in his life.

For the first time in his life, the possibilities were truly endless. That day changed his life forever. Timmy Johnston would never be the same.

23

No More Dieting

"Morning Timmy, how is your week going so far?" Matthew asked at their Wednesday meeting.

"Well Matthew, this week has flown by. I have been thinking about our meeting since our emails on Sunday."

"I was excited by your email, as it showed a sense of purpose and commitment. Yet I was also curious as to what happened on Saturday. Do you remember seeing me when you were leaving the game?"

"No, I don't remember seeing you."

"I woke up late Sunday morning and Jason was gone. He left a note, I cleaned up the house, and I emailed you."

"Do you want to tell me about what happened on Saturday? You don't have to if you don't want. On the way out when I saw Jason, he said you were happy and doing great, then he came back from the concession stand and you were a different person."

"Sure, I will tell you about it."

Timmy went on to tell Matthew what had happened. He told him about the amazing feeling he had, and how it was dashed when he realized that she was waving at some guy behind him. He told Matthew that he vowed to change his life so that he would not be alone, but also be with a girl of that caliber.

"I understand. Not just how you felt, but why that is such a powerful motivator. The thing is, you can meet a great woman just the way you are now; you just aren't ready yet."

"Yeah, right! Only a girl close to my size would be interested in me. NO way a girl like Natalie is going to go for a guy over 300 pounds."

"Wait a second, are you talking about Natalie Williams? Is that the girl you were talking about?"

Timmy looked up with a grin on his face that is unmistakable. He looks like a little kid in a candy store. "Yes, that is the one."

"Ok, this makes much more sense now. I am a decade out of college, I am only here part-time, and I know who you are talking about.

"So you want Natalie, or a girl like her?"

"Yes, but more importantly I don't want to end up alone. I want to be sociable and have friends like so many people I saw at the football game."

"Well, if that is the case, then we have some work to do."

"I know," replied Timmy. "I understand that a beautiful woman like that has her choice of men to pick from, and it makes sense why she was blowing kisses to the guy behind me. Heck, he reminded me of a younger version of you, Matthew."

Chuckling out loud, Matthew said, "Thanks for the compliment, but trust me, there are way more important things than just looks and beauty. You have a lot to offer a woman, Timmy. You are smart, dedicated, and have a heart of gold.

"What is really holding you back is that no woman is going to believe in you until YOU believe in you. You don't have to wait until you are 180 pounds to meet women, but you do have to believe in yourself to meet women."

"I hear you, Matthew, but it is just hard for me because I am so conscious of my weight. I think it will really help my confidence when I start seeing the weight come off. It was great that my brother saw a difference, but I am ready to do whatever it takes to lose the next 100 pounds."

"If you want it bad enough, I can definitely help you.

"I am excited to see that you are motivated to do this, but part of me hopes you aren't doing this for just a girl."

"Oh no, Matthew! I don't want you to think that. I want to lose the weight so I don't end up alone, or in the hospital like my mom. I want to live a long healthy life…but I want to do it as quickly as possible because I don't want to be overweight my entire time in college.

"I saw all these people having fun, hanging out, and throwing the football in the parking lot. I can't do those things right now. Sure, the whole Natalie thing is part of it, but I think that was just the tipping point for me."

"That's good to hear. I figured there had to be more than just a girl."

"It is, trust me. I want to do the things college kids do, and because I can't, it hurts my self-confidence even more."

Matthew put his arm around Timmy. "it takes a real man to admit what you just did. I know that wasn't easy to do. Don't worry; I am going to help you reach your goal. You put in the effort and I give you my word that you will get where you want to go."

"Thanks, Matthew. I don't want to waste another second. Can we get started? I want to have one of those big days where I learn a lot and take a lot of notes. Not to mention I gained seven pounds over the weekend."

"Hold on a second. You gained seven pounds?"

"That is what the scale said on Sunday. I was doing so well, but I know I drank beer and ate some hot dogs at the game. When I woke up Sunday morning, there were two empty pizza boxes, but I can't remember if I even ate any. I think it is safe to say I did."

"Stop right there. Don't worry about it one bit. There is no way you put on seven pounds of fat. It isn't possible to put on that much fat in such a short period of time. Your weight gain can be attributed to water weight. Alcohol and the sodium in the hot dogs and pizza are causing you to retain water. Just keep drinking water and doing what you have been doing. When is the last time you weighed yourself?"

"Sunday morning."

"Ok, good. Wait until Sunday if you can, or even tomorrow morning if you can't wait. When you step on the scale, I think you will see that most of that weight is already gone. So don't sweat it. You didn't undo six weeks worth of work in one day.

"This will make more sense as we discuss how the body works. You will see the difference between fat and water weight and why you shouldn't worry about this."

"Sounds good to me! I trust you," said Timmy.

"Great, now let's get cracking!

"You are already making great progress with the four basics, which are?"

"Walking, water, portion control, and The Squeeze," responded Timmy.

"Exactly. Now it's time to take things up a notch. It is great that you are watching your portions, but now we are going to take things to the next level. To do this, we are going to focus on nutrition."

"Nutrition? Why can't you teach me some new exercises first?"

"I could do that," replied Matthew, "but you can't exercise your way out of a bad diet.

"Yeah, go ahead. Write that down in big letters on the top of your page."

"Let me guess, the sooner I start eating healthier, the faster I will get results?"

"You got it! I want to ask you a question. How do you feel when you hear the word 'diet?'"

Timmy's eyes rolled around in his head as if to say, "Oh great, here we go again…"

Matthew chuckled. "I bet a blind man could have read the expression on your face."

"Diets…really? I was hoping you had something better in store for me."

"Well, let me tell you something; I hate diets! I hate what the word has come to mean. There is a reason it is spelled that way, because most people would rather D-I-E than D-I-E-T!

"I don't know what it is, but something about that word just makes people cringe. It makes people feel like they have to sacrifice things they love and enjoy."

"Diets stink. Mom always hated them."

"I understand where she is coming from. It seems that all 'diets' seem to be tied to a time scale. The ten day diet, the one month diet, the 'don't eat this for three months' diet. Whatever it is."

"Yeah, Mom would always start out good for a few days, sometimes a few weeks, but ultimately she would be back where she started."

"That is how it happens, Timmy. Ever wonder where the term 'yo-yo dieting' came from?"

"I have heard that before, but I didn't know what it had to do with dieting. I had a yo-yo as a kid, and that is what I would always think about."

"That's funny. I was pretty good at the yo-yo myself. Used to do it to kill time at swim meets as a kid. But yo-yo dieting goes a little something like this. Let's just assume you go on a diet for let's say six weeks and you lose 10 pounds. That is great. But then you stop the diet and go back to your old habits. What do you think is going to happen?"

"Well, if you stop what you were doing to lose the weight, you are going to put it back on, right?"

"Exactly!

"Just like a 'yo-yo,' your weight went d-o-w-n and then when you stopped the diet and went back to the old habits, your weight went back u-p!

"Diet…lose weight. Return to old habits…gain weight back. New diet…lose weight. Return to hold habits…gain weight back. A newer diet… you get the picture."

Timmy chuckled out loud. "That's pretty funny! And simple to understand, too!" The smile then melted from his face and Timmy's demeanor changed as he realized that his mom was that person, the "yo-yo dieter."

"Mom was that person for years," said a solemn Timmy. "I hated seeing her so frustrated. She would try so hard, then I don't know what would happen, but she would always go back to the way she was."

"I know, Timmy. It is very hard. Not only is it hard to be the person on the diet, but also it is hard to watch the people you love and care about stumble on their diets."

"Yeah, Mom took things pretty hard sometimes, especially when the weight came back on."

"I have some good news for you though."

"Oh really, what is that? Doesn't seem like there could be much good news to dieting."

"Let's get one thing straight, what I am about to teach you is NOT a diet! I am not about diets, and living a Lean Life is not about dieting!"

"Then what are you about?"

"I am about living a lifestyle with sound nutritional habits so that there is no need to diet. By living life this way, and making certain habits a part of you, there will never be a need to 'DIE-t.'"

"That makes sense. But what about a diet where you lose lots of weight fast, and then you just maintain?"

"That is wishful thinking, Timmy. I hate to say it, but there will NEVER be a diet you can do for a fixed amount of time that will continue to work when you stop the diet. Does that make sense?"

"It is starting to sink in. So what you are saying is that no matter what amazing 'diet' you try, if you go back to your old ways, you will put the weight back on and become a yo-yo dieter."

"Exactly. If you want to get that trimmer, leaner, sexy body…and keep it, then you need to get good habits, maintain them, and make it a part of your life!

"Besides, if you lose the weight too fast, your skin can't keep up and you will end up being skinny with a lot of extra skin hanging around. Then the only thing that can help you is surgery."

"I never thought about that."

"Yes, it's true. That is why it is important to lose weight in a healthy manner and drink lots of water when you do it as it helps with the elasticity of your skin."

"Makes sense to me!"

Matthew saw the excitement building on Timmy's face and in his body language, so in his best 'infomercial voice' he said, "Are you ready to ditch dieting forever? Are you ready to stop starving yourself? Are you ready for something that really works?

"If you answered YES to any of those questions, then let's take a five minute break so we can get started!"

Timmy almost fell out of his chair laughing at Matthew.

"I'm glad you have a sense of humor. I'm going to take that break and come back ready to learn."

Still laughing, Matthew said, "Great, see you back here in five."

24

Starving Yourself Doesn't Work

"I was just watching you walk down the hall, and I can tell you have really been working on your posture. Not only are your feet pointing more straight ahead, but it looks like your shoes are wearing better."

"Thanks for noticing, Matthew. I can tell a difference when I walk, but the thing where I definitely know I am making a difference is when I look at my shoes. I am totally blown away that my shoes are wearing so well. I have been walking more than I ever have in my life, and I can still wear the shoes. They are only worn on a slight angle, not the way they used to be."

"That is great, Timmy. You have come a long way in a short period of time. You are turning back years of bad posture little by little. All those little things you are doing on a daily bases ARE making a big difference."

"I have to say, I am pleasantly surprised that my shoes aren't wearing as bad and as fast as they used to. I know it will be even better as I keep losing weight. I know I am putting a lot of strain in my shoes. But enough about my shoes, I'm ready to learn about nutrition."

"Then let's get started.

"Before we just dive into a nutritional plan, I think it is a good idea to take a little time and explain a little bit about the body and how it works. I believe that if you know and understand a bit about how the body works and the science behind it, it will be easier for you to make the nutritional plan work for you.

"How would you like it if I taught you a way to eat that doesn't rely on constant self-control, but naturally tells your body to stop eating? Imagine eating meals where you feel full and satisfied, yet you are losing lots of unwanted body fat. How does that sound?"

Timmy's demeanor changed. "I would say that sounds great, but it also sounds pretty complex. I usually get lost when things get all complex and scientific."

"I am the same way. Don't worry; I am going to keep this pretty simple. Feel free to stop me anytime if you have questions or need me to go over something."

"Sounds good!"

"Let's start with a quick question. Do you know the three types of macronutrients that make up the food we eat?"

"Macronutrients…not two seconds ago you said this wasn't going to be too scientific!"

Chuckling, Matthew continued. "Let me give you a hint; you probably look for them on the 'nutrition info' panel that is on almost all foods that we eat."

Timmy sarcastically says, "Do I look like I have read a lot of nutrition info? I mean, I know what the label is, but I don't know how to make sense of it all."

"That is great. Thanks for telling me. I want you to get this stuff, so we will cover how to read a nutrition label. For right now though, I just want to touch on the label, and we will go into more depth a little bit later. Will that work for you?"

"Sure. I am sure you have a reason behind your madness."

Matthew laughs, "I like to think I do."

He then goes to his desk and picks up a label he ripped off of a box of crackers from the teachers' lounge.

Nutrition Facts

Serving Size 5 Crackers (16g)
Servings Per Container About 28

Amount Per Serving

Calories 80 Calories from Fat 40

	% Daily Value*
Total Fat 4.5g	**7%**
Saturated Fat 1g	**5%**
Trans Fat 0g	
Polyunsaturated Fat 1.5g	
Monounsaturated Fat 2g	
Cholesterol 0mg	**0%**
Sodium 140mg	**6%**
Total Carbohydrate 9g	**3%**
Dietary Fiber less than 1g	**1%**
Sugars 1g	
Protein 1g	

Vitamin A 0% • Vitamin C 0%
Calcium 0% • Iron 2%

*Percent Daily Values are based on a 2,000 calorie diet. Your daily values may be higher or lower depending on your calorie needs:

	Calories	2,000	2,500
Total Fat	Less than	65g	80g
Sat Fat	Less than	20g	25g
Cholesterol	Less than	300mg	300mg
Sodium	Less than	2,400mg	2,400mg
Total Carbohydrate		300g	375g
Dietary Fiber		25g	30g

"There is a lot of information on the nutritional label, but there are only three macronutrients. Those are fats, proteins, and carbohydrates."

"Oh that is what you were asking? I knew that, I just didn't know they were called macronutrients."

"That is all I was asking about for now. But here is a bonus question for you since you know what fats, protein, and carbohydrates are. Do you know how many calories are in a gram of each one?"

Timmy rolled his eyes. "Argh. My mom hated counting calories, and that is what you are having me do now."

"Nope, not at all. Before you get all worked up, give me a minute.

"I am teaching you to live a healthy lifestyle and one that doesn't revolve around counting calories. I just want you to know this information, as it will be important for what we are going to cover very shortly."

"Ok. Fine."

"It is pretty easy. A gram of fat has 9 calories per gram, and protein and carbohydrates each have 4 calories per gram."

"Wait a second. A gram is a gram right? So the same gram of fat has more than twice the calories of carbohydrates or protein?"

"You nailed it. The whole point of that question was for you to see that a gram of fat has more than twice the 'energy' as a gram of carbs or protein. This means that gram for gram, fat is the most efficient source of energy for the body."

"Hold on a sec. What are 'carbs?'"

"Oh sorry, carbs is just a shorter term for carbohydrates."

"Ok, that is what I thought."

"So let me see if I have this straight. Fat is the most efficient source of energy because gram for gram, it has more calories, or energy, than carbs or protein."

"That's it. That is all I wanted you to understand at this point. We will go into more depth later. But you need to understand that fact to understand how the body works. Now, are you ready to take a trip?"

"Sure, where are we going?" Timmy asked as his face lit up.

"We are going to go back several hundred years to the caveman days. We are going back to a time before there were grocery stores and you only ate what you picked in the wild, or killed."

"Psssh. I thought we were going on a field trip to the grocery store or something."

Matthew didn't let Timmy's sarcastic comment faze him. He kept on going.

"You can probably imagine that finding food was quite a bit tougher back then. There were no stores, no restaurants, no seven-elevens. In fact, finding food was a full-time job back then.

"Depending on the season, or geographical location, it could be very hard to pick something off the land to eat. Can you image trying to pick berries, or anything to eat for that matter, when it is covered under three feet of snow?"

"I never really thought of it like that."

"Exactly. It isn't happening. If there is three feet of snow on the ground, it is also going to be harder to find animals, as they feed off those same berries and plants. Not to mention lots of animals go into hibernation or relocate during the winter. If it is hard for the animals to find something to eat, you can bet it would certainly be hard for the humans to find something to eat as well."

"That's great, Matthew, but what does this have to do with anything?"

"Well, let me tell you.

"Since the cavemen didn't always know when their next meal was coming, and they might only eat one time per day, or sometimes only once in a few days, as a survival mechanism, their bodies would try to preserve body fat.

"Not only does the body fat provide warmth, but as we stated earlier…"

Timmy interrupted, "It is the body's most efficient fuel source!"

"Exactly.

"Did your mom ever say anything like 'I can't eat anything for the rest of the day, or the next few days because I want to look good this weekend in my dress, for the wedding, for the party, or anything like that?"

"I do remember her doing that, but it was years ago when she and Dad were a lot more social. It was before Dad lost his job and all."

"Yeah, a lot of people have done it, and the reason I asked about your mom is that it is something that is more common with women than with men. Women are more likely to do something related with starving themselves, whereas the men are more likely to try anything to help with putting on muscle; and I do mean anything.

"You see, your mom figured that not eating would the best way to lose a few pounds and get ready for whatever event she was going to go to with your father."

"Makes sense to me. Not eating much for a day or so sounds like a good way to burn some fat and lose some weight."

"I know, Timmy, it 'sounds' good, but let's take a look at how the body works and see if that holds true.

"Back to our caveman again. As we have already established, nature's way of protecting the caveman was to preserve the body's most efficient fuel source--body fat. Let's take a look at how this happens and why starvation type diets don't work."

"You really like raining on my parade, don't you Matthew? So much of what I thought I knew about the body is turning out to be incorrect."

"It's ok, Timmy. You are not alone. There is so much misinformation out there, most of which originated from quick fixes, so there are a lot of people that have bad or incorrect habits. But like I said earlier, it is never too late to turn it around.

"We have already established that to protect the cavemen, the body liked to preserve body fat as it is the most efficient fuel source, as well as a source of warmth. Here is the kicker. When you go on starvation or very low-calorie type diets, the body shuts down burning fat as a fuel source."

Timmy had a look of disappointment on his face.

"Yes, here is what happens when you do those 'starvation' type diets. First, your body burns up all of the energy that is currently in the digestive system."

"Then it starts burning fat?" chirped an optimistic Timmy.

"Not exactly.

"Once the body burns what is currently in the digestive system, it starts burning your muscles for energy."

"Wait, so are telling me that when you don't eat for a while, your body burns muscle before fat?"

"Pretty much. The body burns the glycogen in your muscles. Before you think I am getting too scientific again, think of glycogen as a sponge that is the fuel for your muscles. Scientifically, glycogen is the carbohydrate stored in the muscles."

"Why is glycogen like a sponge?"

"Great question. I like to use the sponge analogy as I have found that it really helps people understand this concept. I like to think of glycogen like a sponge because glycogen stored in your muscles holds about three to four times its weight in water."

"I get it. A sponge holds water by your sink, and glycogen holds water in your muscles."

Matthew chuckled. "Basically, yes.

"When your body uses this glycogen for energy, it is like burning up your sponge. If you burn up your sponge, there is nothing to hold that water in the muscles any longer and it is excreted from your body."

"This lost water is why so many people 'think' they are losing weight when they do a one day 'starvation' type diet. By depleting their glycogen stores, they can easily lose a few pounds of water weight on the first day."

"Wow. That makes sense because Mom would always be happy with her one-day weight loss. I distinctly remember her doing it because she would still cook for the family but just wouldn't eat anything."

"I have an example of something that happened to me several years ago when I was still in the military. I went through SERE training, which stands for Survival, Evasion, Resistance, and Escape. The training was two weeks. One week of classroom, and then a week of realistic outdoor training where you basically go a week without food."

"You went a week without food? That's what I need right now! I would definitely lose some weight then."

"Not so fast, Timmy. Stay with me.

"I had been working out pretty hard before I even knew I was going to be doing this training, so I was already pretty lean. During the classroom part, a couple of the guys were saying how they were looking forward to 'losing some weight' during the following week. They thought they were going to lose a fair amount of body fat and be ready to hit the beach for summer."

"I'm sure with a week of starvation, they lost a lot of weight."

"Let's take a look at what actually happened at the end of the week. Most of the guys that were hoping to lose several pounds of body fat didn't have any extra lean mass. When I say lean mass, I am talking about muscles. They were just 'normal' guys. These normal guys carrying around extra body fat lost about six to eight pounds on average."

"That doesn't sound too bad, losing six to eight pounds in a week. I lost about twice that, but it took me six weeks!"

"Hold on, Timmy. On the other hand, I was already pretty lean. Do you want to guess how much weight I lost that week?"

"I don't know. Because you were so lean, you probably lost three to five pounds because you didn't have as much fat to lose."

"Is that your final answer?" said Matthew in his best Regis Philbin accent.

Timmy laughed, "Yes, final answer."

"You won't believe this, but I lost almost fifteen pounds during that same week!"

"What? How could that be? It doesn't make sense."

"Let me explain. Because I had been active and working out since I was a child, I had more muscle mass than the other guys. My muscles were full of glycogen before the week started. As the week went on, my body used that glycogen for energy. When my body burned that glycogen, I didn't have as much sponge to hold water anymore."

"So you were dehydrated then?"

"Not at all. The one thing they made sure of is that we had plenty of water, so dehydration was nothing to worry about."

"I'm not sure if I'm getting it."

"That's ok. Remember what I said earlier about burning the glycogen for energy, and that glycogen is like a sponge that holds water?"

"Yes."

"Well, I was completely hydrated, I just didn't have as much 'sponge' or glycogen in my muscles to hold water anymore.

"Let's say we had a sponge that is soaking wet. We will use that to represent being hydrated. Then let's take a pair of scissors, cut the sponge in half, and remove one of the halves."

"Ok, I'm with you."

"Is that sponge that is left still hydrated?"

"Of course, you didn't remove water from the sponge; you just took away part of the sponge."

"Exactly. Same thing happens in your muscles. Instead of scissors cutting and removing the sponge, your body just used it for energy."

Timmy lights up, "I got it! Makes total sense now."

"Great, but do you want to know what was really crazy?"

"What?"

"I gained over twelve pounds back in the first forty-eight hours!"

"How can that be?" asked Timmy with big look of confusion on his face.

"Once that week was over and I could eat again, my first meal, which was actually three meals, was a trip to a Mexican take-out restaurant in San Diego. I ordered chicken nachos with guacamole, a chicken quesadilla, and chicken enchiladas. Each one in its own white, full-size Styrofoam box."

"That is a lot of food!"

"Yes it is. All my friends said I would never be able to eat it because my stomach was supposed to shrink. I don't know what the deal was for me, but aside from sharing some of the nachos, I had no problem polishing it all off!

"After eating all of that food, my body processed the carbohydrates to use as immediate energy, but more importantly, those carbohydrates were used by my body to replenish its glycogen stores! So, as my body was replenishing all of the glycogen in my muscles, guess what it needed?"

"I'm not sure."

"Glycogen is like a…"

"Sponge."

"Very good. So if…"

"Water. All that glycogen, which is like a sponge in your muscles, would need water."

"High five for Timmy!"

Both of their hands collided with a resounding SMACK!

"That was the other interesting thing. I was drinking lots of water, but I wasn't really going to the bathroom very much."

Timmy gave Matthew a puzzled look.

"I wasn't going to the restroom because I had replenished the 'sponge,' or glycogen, in my muscles, and that sponge was absorbing a majority of the water I was drinking.

"When I was burning up my glycogen, my body had to process that extra water. Now I was refilling my glycogen stores, and my body needed to absorb all the water it could.

"Most of the fluids I drank for those first two days went into my muscles as I gained a majority of my weight back very rapidly. This only happens because it was water weight, not fat weight."

"That makes sense. Every time Mom did one of her little starvation diets, I always remember her saying how she put the weight back on as fast as she took it off."

"She was just like you during SERE school. She was losing water weight by not eating, but once she ate her biscuits, pancakes, and French toast, she replenished her glycogen stores and put the water weight back on. She was losing weight, but she wasn't losing body fat."

"It is great that you understand this concept. Now you can see that your losing fiftenn pounds of fat over six weeks is a much better long-term result than if you had just starved yourself over a weekend to lose five pounds of water weight.

"Not only that, but you now have the knowledge and ability to help and teach others about why starvation diets don't work."

"I like that. Definitely going to talk to Mom about this."

"That wasn't too hard or scientific now was it?"

"Not at all. You made it pretty straightforward and easy to understand."

"That is the goal for what we are doing here. I do want to say that it was kept basic for a reason. I wanted to keep it simple so you would grasp the concept. I don't want you to think that I taught you everything there is to know about how the body works.

"My goal is to present you with the core information in a way that you understand it for the purpose of dispelling many of the 'diet myths' that are out there."

"I understand, Matthew. I know there are complex steps in those processes, but I'm glad you kept it simple. So what's next?"

"I'm glad you asked. I figured we could take another quick break to stretch and get some water, then keep moving on.

"Since we just discussed how starvation type diets don't burn fat, I figured the next thing we could talk about is how to really get your body in a fat-burning process."

"Now we're talking!" Timmy stood up to do The Squeeze. "Let's make this a quick break so we can keep going."

"Fine, see you back here in 3 minutes!" Matthew said, as they both briskly left the office and headed towards the restroom.

25

Be a Fat-Burning Machine

"Now that I have shown you how and why starvation 'diets' don't work, are you ready to learn how you can turn your body into a fat burning machine?"

"You bet," exclaimed Timmy.

"Just as you couldn't believe that not eating wasn't a good way to lose weight, I bet you are going to have a hard time believing that you can eat five or six times per day and really burn some fat!"

Timmy laughs. "Normally I would be skeptical, but you have shown me that you are full of surprises."

"I can sense you questioning me a bit here. Notice I said you can eat six times per day, but I didn't say you could eat triple cheeseburgers and fries six times a day."

"Very funny, Matthew. I figured that much."

"Just keeping you on your toes, Timmy. You're not the only one that can be sarcastic every now and then you know," said Matthew with a smirk on his face.

"As I have been saying, The Lean Life is about adopting some sound nutritional principals and applying them to your life.

"Here is one of the core principles. You should be eating about every three hours throughout the day."

"Really?" said Timmy with a look of uncertainty on his face. "I want to believe you, but I'm still having a hard time with the fact that most of what you are telling me flies in the face of everything I have done my entire life."

"I completely understand. I know it is hard when in your entire life you have been told to eat only three meals per day, that snacking is bad, and a host of other things that are based on old knowledge and haven't been updated in many years.

"Seek out people that are in good shape and ask them what they do. You don't have to take just my word for it."

"No, no. That isn't what I'm saying. It's just tough when you start to realize you have been doing it all 'wrong' for so long."

"Put all of that in the past. Make changes today, in the present, that will give you the future that you want.

"Let's get back to our caveman because I think it will be easier for you to 'digest' the idea of eating six times per day once you learn the reasons and science behind it."

"You do seem to have a knack for having it all make sense."

"Earlier when we talked about the caveman we learned that the body wanted to 'hold on' to body fat when it wasn't being fed regularly.

"What do you think your body wants to do with body fat when it knows it is getting fed multiple times per day?"

"I know you want me to say that it is going to burn fat, but if you are eating more times per day, won't you gain more weight?"

"Great question. Let's look at this a bit more.

"First, when you are eating multiple times per day, you won't get those big hunger pains or that 'I'm starving' feeling that usually leads to overeating.

"Second, when you start feeding your body every three hours consistently, it realizes it doesn't need to maintain all this extra energy, which in this case is stored body fat. The body goes, 'hmm…I get fed good energy every few hours. It is a lot more work and effort to carry all this extra stored energy around, so I think I can start letting some of it go.'"

"That sounds good, Matthew, but how long does it take for that to start happening?"

"Great question. Here is the deal. Like most people, I am sure you haven't eaten this way in a long time, if ever, in your life. So don't think you can spend years and years of not feeding your body properly, make these changes, and your body is going to 'believe' it after only a few days.

"It will take a little bit of time for your body to realize, 'Hey, this isn't a fluke.' It usually takes a few weeks, but your body will realize that it is being provided good nutrition and energy multiple times per day and will in turn start to burn some of those excess energy reserves, which we know to be body fat."

"It sounds so simple. But why have we been told since we were kids to eat only three meals per day?"

"I wish I had a good answer for you on that, but I don't. I can't control what the government tells people to do. I can tell you that if you want to lose body fat and get lean, eating three meals per day is not the best or most efficient way to get there."

Timmy had a puzzled look on his face.

"What is it, Timmy? I can see that something is still bothering you."

"Yes. You are saying to eat five to six meals per day, but what do you mean by a meal, and when do I eat all of these meals? It sounds like a lot of work, a lot of time, and a lot of money to eat that way."

"Excellent question. Let me cover when to eat them first, as that is easier to answer. Basically, you will eat your breakfast, lunch, and dinner. But you will be adding a mini-meal or snack between lunch and dinner, and another one after dinner, closer to bedtime. So that will give you five meals for the day."

"What about the sixth meal?"

"Great question. If you are up early in the morning so there are five or more hours between when you first get up until the time when you eat lunch, then add a mini-meal or snack between breakfast and lunch."

"Ok, so this is really pretty easy then. I am basically adding two or three mini-meals or snacks to my regular meals."

"Yup. It is that easy."

"Ok, now what goes into those meals?"

"When I say 'meal,' I don't mean throwing out the white tablecloth and having multiple courses. For our purposes, the definition of a 'meal' will be very basic. We will get into this in more detail later, but for now, a meal will be considered any time we consume food."

"What about mini-meals or snacks?"

"Those are just going to be smaller versions of full meals.

"Just so you aren't confused…" Matthew opened his desk and pulled out a zip-lock baggie with a few almonds, some raisins, and four Triscuits with peanut butter in it. "See this food? It is considered a meal, but I have found that calling it a mini-meal or a snack makes it easier for people to understand."

"That is a meal? Doesn't look like very much food, but I will say that it looks pretty easy to eat and carry around."

"Exactly. I'm glad you saw that. It is easy to eat, easy to prepare, and easy to carry around. We will get into what comprises a meal a little bit later, but I just wanted to show you this example of one of my meals for today."

"How many meals to you typically eat per day, Matthew?"

"I typically eat six times per day. If I am on the road or working eighteen plus hour days, I might eat closer to seven or eight times. For the way you and most others will look at this right now, it seems like a lot. To put this in context, I probably eat two to three of what most people would consider small 'meals,' with the other 'meals' being what you would consider 'snacks' or what I like to call mini-meals.

"Again, we will get into more depth as far as what we should be eating in these meals, but just know that when you are eating five or six times per day, your meals will be smaller."

"Your snack actually looks pretty good. I am looking forward to changing my habits and seeing if it will help me lose weight faster. I am just worried about being hungry."

"That is a great attitude to have. Trust me. In your email on Sunday you said you wanted to take things to the next level. This is a fundamental aspect of doing that. As far as the hunger goes, I think you will be surprised. I know my little baggie doesn't look like a lot of food, but trust me when I tell you that you will very seldom be hungry when you are eating five or six times per day, even if they are smaller portions than what you are used to."

"Do I still need to eat on salad plates?"

"Why wouldn't you? What I am teaching you now doesn't replace what you learned earlier. Those are the most basic of fundamentals and won't change. You will always want to practice good portion control, move, and drink water.

"I understand your fears and concerns. What you will realize after you start eating this way is that you won't ever be 'starving.' You won't get to lunch ready to devour the entire buffet and completely overeat."

Timmy laughed. "I have to admit, there are times that I am so hungry that I think to myself, 'This salad plate just won't cut it. I just want to go through the food line again.'"

"I have been there before many times myself. How would you like to learn a little trick so that when you have those moments of starvation you don't overeat?"

"That would be great! What is it?"

"It takes the body about twenty minutes to register that you are 'full.' So those times when you sit down at the table because you are 'starving' and start shoveling food into your face like you are in a hot-dog eating contest, it will take about twenty minutes for your brain to register that you are 'full' and tell your body to stop eating.

"Do you ever wonder how you get that 'I'm stuffed' feeling? That is how it happens. Your body would have been satisfied with the first five minutes of food you ate, but your brain didn't realize it until the twenty-minute mark. So you ate food for another ten minutes that your body didn't really need."

"I have totally been there! The question is, what can I do about it?"

"Great question. Being aware of how the body works is half the battle. But I would never leave you with just that. There are three big things you can do.

"First, drink a full eight- to twelve-ounce glass of water before your meals. Not only will this help put something in your stomach, but as we discussed earlier, a lot of hunger can be disguised as dehydration. It is best to drink water twenty to thirty minutes before a meal, but even if you have to do it right before the meal, it is better than nothing.

"Second, this might sound very simple, but it is important. Chew your food thoroughly before swallowing. Digestion starts in your mouth with the enzymes that are in your saliva. I know you are hungry, but giving that big bite of pizza only three chews before forcing a swallow is not the way to optimize your digestive process. Chewing your food slowly also helps with our third point.

"The final thing you can do is enjoy your food! Take your time and savor the flavors of the food. By chewing completely and taking your time, you are allowing your body to work properly so that it can naturally send out 'stop eating' signals. I know we are all in a rush, but a few more seconds of chewing goes a long way and isn't going to ruin your day."

"Wait a second, what do you mean 'stop eating' signals?"

"We will cover that more in depth a little bit later. Remember earlier when I said I was going to teach you a way to eat that didn't rely on self-control, but rather let your body naturally tell you to stop eating?"

"Yes, I remember that."

"Well, once we build these fundamentals, I will teach you some very cool natural ways to use your body's hormones to help you eat less and feel satisfied. Just stick with me for a bit."

"Sounds good, Matthew!"

"OK, back to chewing our food.

"Fight the urge to inhale that first slice of pizza. If you do inhale it, that is ok. Pause for a few minutes, drink some water, engage in conversation, and give your body a chance to register what you have already eaten before reaching for another slice. The more time you let pass, the more you give your brain a chance to catch up with your stomach."

BEEP…BEEP…BEEP

Timmy's cell phone went off as he forgot to put it on vibrate.

"You got a call?" asked Matthew.

"No, not at all," replied Timmy. He pulled the phone out of his pocket and showed the screen to Matthew:

'I am a fat-burning machine. People are drawn to me.'

"John told me to do this thing called…"

"Affirmation station. I know. I do the same thing." Matthew had a sly grin on his face and said, "But I do it with my phone on vibrate."

Timmy apologized for the disruption.

"Not a problem," said Matthew, still smiling. "I am glad you are using those tools. They are very effective."

"Now where were we? Oh, that's right.

"Don't make it hard on yourself by having to use your discipline to stop eating. Let the body do it for you naturally. Trust me; you won't feel deprived. In fact, you will feel pretty satisfied when you let the body work the way it was intended."

Timmy looked at the ground, shaking his head. "That pizza story really hits home. That is pretty much how I ate for years. I would be starving and eat four or five slices of pizza before I would even pause to take a drink. People would kid me and say 'breathe' while I was eating."

"I have been the same way as well," said Matthew.

"The thing is, I would feel stuffed every single time. I figured that was just my body. I would be starving one minute and completely stuffed the next. I had no idea how to eat to be satisfied."

"I too look back on my eating habits earlier in life, and they were not the greatest. I would eat twenty plus pieces of pizza after a swim practice and be stuffed for hours until the next one. The only thing that saved me was the amount of exercise I was doing. But we all know that can't last forever."

"And that you can't exercise your way out of a bad diet," chimed in Timmy with a smile.

Matthew laughed.

"As I got older and wasn't exercising five hours a day, I saw that I had to make changes. That is the beauty of understanding the body and how it works.

"I will be the first to admit, I am not very good at relying on will power and commitment as ways to curb my eating. I can do it for the short-term, but not the long-term. That is why I like to make it easier by letting my body do its job. That way I am not relying on just my will power to not eat that next slice of pizza, or grab dessert."

"You ARE human," joked Timmy.

"Very much so. Even though people look at me and think differently."

"I can't wait to try these new eating habits. I am excited about the possibility of not being starving before each meal, and it is nice to know that if it does happen, I will know how to deal with it so that I don't over eat.

"I have to admit, it has been tough sometimes to use the salad plate. I fight going back for seconds, but I have been known to kind of pile it a bit higher than usual."

"That is perfectly normal, Timmy. It is better for you to pile a salad plate a little bit higher than it is to eat an entire dinner-sized plate, that's for sure. Just keep doing what you have been doing. The weight is definitely coming off; you just have to stick with it."

"You don't have to worry about me sticking with it," replied Timmy.

"That said--I know you said we are going to talk about it--the only thing I am wondering right now is what to eat. The cafeteria only serves three meals per day, so I don't know what to do for the other three or more meals in the day."

"I like where your head is at. Those are great questions and it shows you are really getting this material and want to make a change."

Matthew threw the zip-lock baggie to Timmy.

"Go ahead and eat this while I talk. I made it for you."

"Thanks, Matthew!"

"That will be your second meal of the day and it isn't even lunch time yet."

Timmy smiled and nodded, but he can't talk because he already has a mouth full of food.

"I figured the best thing to do right now was for me just to give you a few ideas for snacks that you can use for the next few days until we meet again. At that time, we will go over fats/carbs/protein in depth so you will then be able to build your own tasty meals."

Timmy took his time chewing before swallowing. "That sounds great, Matthew. If you can give me a few meal ideas, that would be great."

"You are in luck, Timmy."

Matthew reached under his desk and pulled out a small, collapsible, blue cooler with two zippers on it.

"I put this together for you to keep. I use one every day and it really helps make it easier. You can just put it in your backpack and carry it around with you during the day, or take it with you on weekends."

Timmy lit up. "Thanks Matthew!"

Matthew unzipped the side pocket and pulled out a Ziploc baggie. "Here is a good little snack."

The baggie had five or six almonds in it, along with four Triscuits made into two sandwiches with peanut butter. There were two other baggies, one with just almonds in it, another with just Triscuits, and a third bag with some sort of powder.

Matthew then unzipped the main compartment, where he pulled out a small ice pack, followed by some 2% Greek yogurt, low-fat cottage cheese, a small jar of organic peanut butter, and an apple.

"I want you to have these things to get started," said Matthew.

"Next week we will learn all about these types of foods so that you can make your own healthy snacks and meals.

"For now, we just want to keep things simple. For the next week, each time you have a snack, I want it to have five or six almonds, four Triscuits with peanut butter, and a couple of teaspoons of yogurt or cottage cheese.

"When you eat the apple, I want you to eat six to eight almonds with it, OR put the organic peanut butter on the slices. You will also have a couple of spoonfuls of either the yogurt or the cottage cheese."

"That sounds easy enough. What is that powder?"

"That is just 100% whey protein powder."

Timmy made a funny face and was about to speak when Matthew spoke first...

"I know what you are probably thinking. That protein powders are gross and only for bodybuilders."

Timmy slightly nodded his head.

"That is just an old stereotype. Protein powders have come a LONG way over the past few years in taste and in mixing ability. So don't let that old, tired story hold you back. The toughest thing for people to get in their diet is protein. It just isn't 'easily' available, especially without preparation or being refrigerated. Next week we are going to learn all about protein, but for now there will be times when having yogurt or cottage cheese easily available isn't going to be an option. With this little baggie of protein powder, you have something you can take with you wherever you go and easily mix it with water."

Timmy looked up at Matthew, "Do you actually like the protein powder, or is it just something you are telling me to do?"

Chuckling out loud. "I actually use the protein powder all the time. It isn't always easy to get 'real food' sources of protein, so I always have a baggie of protein with me. Trust me; I am all about making this as easy as possible.

"I know you are probably worried about the taste as well. Protein powders have come a long way. Whey mixes almost instantly with water, and it actually tastes great."

Timmy doesn't look completely convinced.

"See the size of this scoop?" Matthew held up the little plastic piece. "This one scoop has the same amount of protein as an entire chicken breast, or about four eggs."

Timmy's eyes got really big.

"Exactly. That is why I use the powder. I try to eat my protein in whole food form as much as I can, but when eating six times per day, I find it helps me out to be able to get quality protein so quickly and easily."

"Wait a second; is that what you are often drinking during our meetings? I thought it looked like a fruit juice or something."

"You guessed it!"

"That makes me feel good to know that you take the protein powder."

"I sure do. One thing you will learn about me is that I practice what I preach. I won't be telling you stuff that I don't do myself."

"I really like that," said a comforted Timmy.

"We got a little ahead of ourselves with the protein powder, and I was even hesitant to bring it up now, but I figured you could handle it. We will get into everything in more depth next week."

Matthew put everything back in the cooler, zipped it up, and handed it to Timmy. "See you next week, and let me know if you have any questions along the way.

"After next week, you will know how to read a food label and how to pick good foods to eat."

"I am looking forward it! I have noticed one thing already. It is almost time for lunch, and I don't feel like gnawing my own arm off because I am so hungry. That little 'meal' is already making a difference. It is going to be much easier to eat off the salad plate today."

"That is what I like to hear! Have a great rest of the week, and I will see you Wednesday."

Timmy left the office with a spring in his step.

26

Letter to Mom #4 – Speed Bumps and Recovery

Class was finally over and Timmy was looking forward to the walk back to his apartment. Instead of taking the most direct route like he used to do, he now mixes it up to take longer walks and to enjoy the beautiful scenery the campus has to offer.

Not only does he get to see new people, buildings, and things, but also it allows him to clear his head and visualize where he wants to be in life, all while keeping moving.

Today was different than most days. He had learned so much from Matthew this morning, and to think it had only been three days since he sent Matthew an email asking for help with taking things to the next level. Timmy smiled to himself as he really was amazed at how fast his life was turning around.

Timmy left his meeting with Matthew with a new cooler, but more importantly with a new sense of understanding. There was still a small part of him that was skeptical, but nothing could stop the sense of excitement as he had to try out this new way of eating. Eating six times per day instead of just three, could it really work?

It didn't matter. Timmy continued walking, visualizing himself losing weight, and eventually arriving at his goal weight of 180 pounds. By making it clear in his mind, he paved the way for his body to follow.

While climbing the steps to his apartment, something clicked in Timmy's head. He had no idea why, but he was dying to step on the scale to see if Matthew was right.

When he burst into his living room, he tossed his belongings aside and headed to the bathroom. Timmy stood there staring at the scale for a moment.

"Matthew said to wait until at least tomorrow, but I just have to see if he is right," thought Timmy to himself.

He stood there for another minute before slowly stepping onto the scale. Much to his surprise, he had already lost five of those seven pounds again.

Timmy knew that Matthew was right again. Sure, he had told him to wait, but this gave him even more confidence.

He moved directly in front of the mirror, placed both hands on the counter and looked intensely at himself in the mirror. "Maybe I owe it to myself to put my stories and bad habits aside, and to fully embrace what he is telling me. He hasn't let me down yet," said Timmy out loud.

He could feel the motivation start to burn in the pit of his gut. "This is a great feeling," he thought to himself. I need to not only keep this going but share it with other people as well.

Timmy grabbed his notebook and a pen and sat on the barstool at the tiny kitchen counter.

Wednesday, October 13

Dear Mom,

I hope I am not interrupting a visualization session, or maybe you are picking this letter up on the way back from a walk. Either way, I am sure you are doing great, especially if you have been putting my letters into action.

All in all, things are going really well. Jason came to visit last weekend for homecoming and we had a great time.

He got in on Friday, and get this, the first thing he noticed when he saw me was that my face looked thinner, and he asked if I had lost weight. You don't know how great a feeling that was!

Mom, I have lost about 15 pounds of fat the right way in only six weeks! Not to mention those new shoes you sent me are wearing normally, and we both know that hasn't happened in years.

I have to tell you Mom; it hasn't all been easy. I had a rough day on Saturday.

Things started out great. Jason and I went to the stadium and we were just hanging out. Then I saw Matthew and brought him over to meet Jason. I think it was really good for Jason to meet him, so he could see that I had good people helping me.

Not to mention that Matthew and John are the ones that got the tickets for us to begin with. So the three of us hung out for a bit and then Matthew had to go. I was kind of feeling the excitement, so Jason and I headed in to find our seats.

We had awesome seats! We were close to the field and all of the activity. We could easily see the cheerleaders, and that is when it happened. Jason went to go grab us some food, and I was just taking it all in: the people, the energy, the excitement.

Then I saw this girl, and she was the most amazing thing I have ever seen in my life. She was one of the cheerleaders down on the field 16 rows in front of us.

You wouldn't believe how she made me light up inside. My stomach came alive, and it felt incredible. I just stood there staring at her. You won't believe this, but she waved at me…or at least I thought she did. That is when things turned for me. I waved back only to realize she was waving at some guy behind me.

Mom, it hurt so badly. It felt like Mike Tyson punched me in the gut after Don King took all my money; that's how bad it hurt. It hit me like a ton of bricks that girls like that don't find fat guys like me attractive. The guy she was waving at was my height, but a lean and muscular 180 pounds or so.

Right after that, Jason came back with food and beer. I just lost it. I chugged an entire beer and ate like three hotdogs in a flash. I ended up having several more beers and ended up having to leave the game before halftime.

The rest of the day was a blur. All I remember is waking up Sunday morning and finding empty pizza boxes and then a note from Jason. I felt like crap. I couldn't even remember if I ate the pizza or not. I just got drunk and apparently I ate a lot too.

I stepped on the scale and it confirmed that I ate way too much. I had gained seven pounds in just a day or so. It was like six week's worth of work was erased on a bad Saturday, or so I thought.

I emailed Matthew and let him know I was ready to make some more changes and take things to the next level. That is where things turned around for me. Our meeting earlier today was amazing!

First off, I learned the difference between fat weight and water weight, as I was so worried that I had gained seven pounds back in that one day. Remember when you used to not eat before special weekends with Dad years ago to lose a few pounds quickly? Well, I learned why that never works, and why you would be frustrated when the pounds came back by the end of the weekend.

All you were losing was water weight, not fat. That is mostly what I gained from my day of drinking beer and salty foods. By mid-week I had lost almost all of the seven pounds already.

I learned the basics of how the body works and why Matthew is having me do things a different way. It was hard at first, because everything he was telling me was different than anything I had ever heard before, but it makes sense.

He told me I should be eating six meals per day. Yeah, I thought it was crazy too, but it isn't. This morning he gave me my own portable cooler full of food. We are going to go more in depth next week, but he gave me several ideas for snacks for now.

I have to say mom, I have already eaten 5 times today, and I feel great. It is really weird. I am not eating a lot of food, but I am not hungry at all! And I actually feel like I have MORE energy!

So that is about it for now. I am going to keep walking, drinking water, eating on salad plates, and doing The Squeeze. I am just going to add in the smaller snacks during the day, which will keep my metabolism going, and help me not be 'starving' when the meals roll around.

I can't wait for you to see the difference! My goal is to be less than 300 pounds by Thanksgiving. And speaking of, don't think for a second I am going to stuff myself silly like I used to do. No need to get a separate ham or turkey for me this year.

Anyway, I have to get some homework done and eat my sixth meal of the day. Take care of yourself, and just know that I love you! Tell everybody I am doing great!

Lil Timmy ☺

27

How to Eat for Fat Loss

Timmy went over to the freezer and pulled out the ice pack and placed it neatly into his cooler. He made sure it was in the middle so that it touched the yogurt, fruit, and cottage cheese he had placed inside.

It hadn't been a full week yet, but Timmy was really enjoying the way he felt when eating six meals a day. He seemed to have consistent energy levels without having any mid-day crashes or being starving at meals.

He was excited for today's meeting with Matthew. Not only to share how well he was feeling, but also because he had a few questions.

Timmy packed the rest of his snacks, grabbed his book bag, and headed out the door.

It was a pleasant fall morning. It was clear, but there was a crisp chill in the air that caused Timmy to zip his jacket. He didn't mind as he really enjoyed walking now. There was just something special about being outside, breathing the fresh air, and being alone with his thoughts.

"Hey Timmy, wait up," came a familiar voice from across the parking lot.

It was Matthew getting his things out of the trunk of his car.

"What are you doing way over here?" inquired Matthew. "Isn't your apartment over there?" he asked as he pointed across campus.

"Yes it is," replied Timmy.

"Then what are you doing all the way over here?" said Matthew with a puzzled look on his face.

"Well, believe it or not, I really enjoy walking. After a while of walking the same direct routes, I wanted some different scenery. Not to mention the fact that the more I walk, the more weight I lose."

"Really?"

"Really."

"Well, what can I say? I am proud of you, Timmy! You really are transforming your life right before your very eyes. The small changes you have made are going to change your life."

"I really am impressed that you are going the extra mile...no pun intended."

"Thanks, Matthew. I would have thought you were crazy if you had told me several weeks ago that not only would I be walking to class, but that I would be walking out of my way to get places, and all the while enjoying it!"

Matthew chuckled.

"I have to drop off a folder for one of the other counselors, so why don't you just meet me up in the office and I will be there in just a minute," said Matthew as they both entered the building.

"Sounds good," replied Timmy as unzipped his jacket and turned towards the water fountain.

Timmy had just placed his stuff on the chair when Matthew arrived at the office.

"I am still blown away at the effort you are putting into your walking, Timmy. You are going to get to your goal weight faster than you think if you keep this up. That said, have you been able to eat six times a day since our last meeting?"

"I sure have. In fact, it has been really easy. I thought it was going to be hard, but it really hasn't been. I even went to the grocery store to get more of the things you gave me."

"How was your trip to the store?"

"It was good, but it was kind of intimidating. The only thing that saved me was that I was only looking for the exact same things you gave me. If I didn't have that, I would have been lost."

"What was intimidating to you?"

"There are just so many options. I know you gave me 2% Greek yogurt, but if you hadn't given me any and just told me to go buy some, I don't know that I would have gotten the right stuff. There was low-fat, no-fat, reduced fat, Greek, regular, plain, and flavored yogurts.

"I tried looking at the nutrition labels, but it was just confusing. Some had high fat, others no fat. Some had more sugar than others. Some yogurts had five lines of ingredients; some just had two or three ingredients total. I had no idea."

"I know how you must have felt. I used to feel the same way until I started learning how to read labels. That is why I wanted to give you food to get started, to make it easier for you."

"It made all the difference in the world. I never thought I would have seen myself eating some of those foods, much less enjoying it!"

"Today you will learn how to read a nutrition label and then you will learn how fats, carbohydrates, and protein fit into your meals. Once you can do those two things, you will no longer be intimidated by the grocery store and you will be able to make your own healthy meals."

"Sounds like a plan to me," said an excited Timmy.

"Again, this can be a very complex subject, but I am going to keep it pretty simple and streamlined. There are a few little secrets that are a bit more advanced, but I think you are ready, so I will throw those in as well."

"I'm ready to learn and take things to the next level. I am really liking the way my body feels, and I know this is just the beginning."

"Great. The first thing we are going to talk about is the three macronutrients in more detail. I think reading the nutritional label will make a lot more sense once you know what you are looking for."

"Yeah, that makes sense. Reading the label isn't that hard; it's understanding what to look for that is hard."

"Exactly. We are going to start by looking at fats, carbs, and protein, the roles they play in the body, and good foods that contain each one. Then we are going to put it all together.

"Before we dive in, I want to take a second to talk about one little scientific thing here. We are going to talk about a hormone in the body called insulin. Insulin basically regulates if the body is going to store fat or burn fat. If your body is producing insulin, you are not burning body fat."

"Ok, simple enough. So how to do I stop my body from producing insulin?"

"You are a fast learner, Timmy. That is exactly what we are going to cover, albeit in a simplified form."

"Simple is better," said Timmy as he turned the page in his notebook, ready to take notes.

"You have probably felt the effects of increased insulin levels."

"Are you sure?"

"Have you ever had a big lunch, usually pizza or pasta, and then a few hours later when you were sitting in class, felt like you couldn't concentrate and that you just wanted to crash?"

"Who hasn't felt that way? Of course I have. I call it my food coma."

Matthew chuckled.

"Is there something wrong with my food coma? It makes for great naps."

"I know it does, as I have taken a quite a few food coma induced naps in my life, but it isn't something you want to do on a daily basis."

"I'm just kidding. I don't really like that. So are you saying insulin is a primary cause of that feeling?"

"You got it. Insulin is also responsible for those times when you have a crazy appetite where you just keep craving food, usually sweets."

"I have definitely had that feeling." Timmy laughs, "Sugar highs and food comas, the story of my life."

Matthew nods in agreement. "I know this is going to sound complex, but it is actually pretty simple. What we want to do is control our insulin levels the best we can. We want to keep things on an even keel and minimize insulin spikes that send our bodies not only into a food coma, but also into the dreaded fat-storing zone."

"I get it. Insulin spikes mean food comas and fat storing, not exactly two things I want to deal with anymore. So what causes the body to produce insulin and insulin spikes?"

"Let's take a look, shall we?

"First, carbohydrates are the primary macronutrient that stimulates the body to produce insulin. Carbohydrates are broken down into a sugar called glucose. This sugar then enters the bloodstream, which in turn raises the blood sugar levels.

"You still with me?"

"Piece of cake. You are making this easy to understand. Keep going."

"Great. This elevated blood sugar triggers the release of insulin, which tells the body to start removing the sugar from the blood stream and storing it.

"Remember earlier when we talked about our sponge?"

"Oh yeah. Glycogen, right?

"That's it. So the body wants to store this sugar as glycogen in the muscles first, but if those glycogen stores are full or there is an excess amount of sugar in the bloodstream, where do you think it is stored?"

"Let me guess. It is stored as body fat?"

"You nailed it. See how easy this is?"

"Ok, so is that why I hear about all these no-carb diets as being popular nowadays? Because no-carb means no insulin production, which means you will burn fat, right?"

"Partly, but the body needs carbohydrates. No-carb only works in the short term as you eventually have to start eating carbs again. Remember, we are about building a lifestyle, so we want to avoid 'diets' and instead build healthy lifelong habits that will help you live a Lean Life."

"That makes sense. I remember reading in my biology class that the brain needed carbohydrates to function, so I can see how no-carbohydrates wouldn't be effective in the long term.

"That said, if carbs are the primary macronutrient that produces insulin, then what do fat and protein do?" asked a very intent Timmy.

"You are on the ball today, I tell you. You keep beating me to my next point!"

Timmy gave Matthew a big smile.

"Let's take a look at fats first. Fats have zero impact on the body as far as producing insulin goes. Fats do perform a very important function though; they slow down absorption of carbohydrates by the body."

Timmy jumped in, "And let me guess, the slower the body gets carbohydrates, the slower it releases insulin, which minimizes the spikes."

"Precisely. Are you sure you didn't study this over the weekend?" said Matthew with a smile.

Timmy just smiled back and said, "So what about protein?"

"You are getting ahead of yourself there. Remember last week when I said I was going to teach you how to eat in such a way that didn't rely just on self-control, and when I said there were going to be a few very important secrets that most people don't know? Well here is one of them.

"When fats hit your stomach, it secretes a hormone that goes directly to the brain that signals the body to STOP EATING."

"Wow, that's pretty cool! Let me make sure I have this straight; fats slow the absorption of carbohydrates in the body, which slows the production of insulin, and fats signal the body to stop eating."

"Exactly. So now you can see the basics of why all those people that ate 'low-fat, high carbohydrate' diets weren't very successful."

Timmy sat there shaking his head. "I remember when Mom was on her 'no fat' kick a few years ago. Everything we had in the house was no-fat or low-fat. It is so funny that I learn about this today. I always wondered why I never got full eating those no-fat crackers, cookies, and other 'healthy' snack foods.

"Now I know. It was partly because there was no fat to tell my brain to stop eating."

"That is part of it. There is another thing that insulin does as well; it makes you feel hungry. So not only do you not feel full when eating all those chips, crackers, and cereal, but the insulin actually makes it so you are hungry to keep eating!

"It has happened to me many times," said Matthew. "You start eating crackers or cereal out of the box and you just keep eating."

"The reason is because there is a delay between the insulin spike and the time until insulin levels decrease. The body has already removed the sugar from the bloodstream, but the insulin is still telling the body it needs more sugar in the bloodstream to process.

"So, the body keeps eating to produce that sugar, even though it doesn't really need to. I don't have to tell you where all of those calories are stored at that point do I?"

Timmy sat there staring off into space and flatly said, "I know, they are stored as body fat."

"You ok, Timmy?"

"Yeah, I am ok. Just thinking of the countless times I have done what you just talked about. I just thought it was normal. I guess it was in my family."

"That is quite all right, Timmy. We can't change the past, but we can make a new beginning, and I think you have already done that."

"I know. Sorry about that. I'm ok. Let's get back to the learning. So what does protein do?"

"I am so glad you are getting this, but I am more impressed with your positive attitude, Timmy. I can tell that you are motivated and that the visualization that John talked with you about is having a positive impact on your life already."

Timmy nodded in agreement, readjusted himself in his chair, and his body language showed that he was engaged again.

"Ok, back to protein.

"Protein has minimal impact on insulin production, but it is very important for another special reason. Protein stimulates another hormone, which produces basically the opposite effect of insulin. Not only does it have the opposite effect, but it helps to control excessive insulin production."

"What is the name of that hormone?" asked Timmy.

"Whoa, I thought you didn't want to get too technical."

"I don't really, but just curious what the hormone opposite of insulin is called."

"The hormone secreted when you consume protein is called glucagon. To keep it simple, insulin tells the body to store blood sugar as glycogen. Glucagon tells the body to release stored glycogen into the system.

"That is about as complex as we need to go right now. Does that make sense?"

"I think so. Mind if I try to recap it all?"

"Go ahead."

"Ok, here goes.

"Insulin determines if your body is storing or burning fat. Carbohydrates stimulate the production of insulin; fats and protein do not. Fats slow the absorption of carbs, which slows the insulin release, and fats signal the brain to tell the body to stop eating."

"Looking good so far."

"Protein secretes a hormone called glucagon that is basically the opposite of insulin, and it helps to manage excessive insulin production.

"What did I miss?"

"You nailed all of the high points. Great job, Timmy!"

"So now that you know the basics about insulin, I am going to show you how to put this into practice on a daily basis."

"Write down this key point. Whenever you have a meal, you want to make sure it contains fats, carbohydrates, and protein. By doing this, you will have pretty good control over your insulin levels.

"The fats will slow the absorption of the carbohydrates into the system, as well as tell the body to stop eating. The protein will secrete a hormone that will keep any insulin spikes in check. The carbs will just do their thing and get broken down into sugar and signal the secretion of insulin."

"The main point is that I shouldn't eat just carbs for a meal, that I should always have fats and protein as well. That is why you told me to eat those snacks the way you did. You wanted to keep it simple, yet make sure I was eating fat and protein with my carbs."

Matthew nodded to Timmy. "Nothing gets by you, does it?"

"Not today it doesn't."

"Good. Now is a good time to take a meal break and use the restroom. When we come back, we will look at each macronutrient individually. This will mean looking at fats, carbs, and protein in more depth, but more importantly, we will go over good foods to eat out of each group.

"How does that sound?"

"Sounds great. This is all really starting to make sense. I can't wait until I am able to build my own healthy meals."

"It won't be long, Timmy; you are almost there!"

"Let's take a break to use the restroom, and then we can come back here and eat our snacks together."

Timmy was already on his feet. "Ready, break!"

Matthew just laughed as Timmy walked out of the office ahead of him. "What a character," he thought to himself.

28

Let's Talk About Fat

"I really like these snacks, or 'mini-meals,' as you like to call them," said Timmy as he and Matthew were eating their second meal of the day.

"Every time I get to a major meal, I am amazed at how I am not starving. Not only does it make the portion control a lot easier, but sometimes I can't believe the small amount of food that actually satisfies me.

"If you had told me a few weeks ago that the smaller meals I have been eating for lunch and dinner would have me satisfied, I probably would have laughed at you."

"I am really glad you are feeling the difference. You approached it with an open mind and the right attitude, and that is why you will get the results. Some people resist it so much that they don't even try it.

"They tell themselves it will never work, so they give up before they start. They let whatever fear they have take control of their mind and they never take action.

"I have worked with some people that were so scared to make the change. They were afraid to succeed, so it took a while to figure out what was holding them back before they could move forward."

"That doesn't make much sense. Why would people be afraid to succeed at something?"

"It doesn't make much sense when you first think about it, but you have to look deeper. Many overweight people have a running story in their head about not being good enough, or that they will never be a normal weight. They have had negative self-talk for so long that they end up believing what the mind tells them.

"So it takes them longer as they first have to change their mindset. Either that, or there is some life event that shocks them into making a change."

"Sort of like my mom's heart attack."

"Exactly. That was your reality check of sorts. Then you got further motivation when you saw how other people were living life at the football game, and you decided then and there that you didn't want to be alone and that you wanted to have friends and eventually a special woman in your life."

"Very true. I have to admit it wasn't easy at first. It was hard for my mind to believe what you were telling me to do. But I did like you said and about a week or so into walking, drinking water, and eating smaller portions it kind of became a part of me. After a month, I honestly couldn't ever see myself eating like I used to.

"Sure, I am not to my goal yet, but I am on my way. I know I have barely scratched the surface, but I wouldn't trade this feeling for anything. Plus, I am becoming more outgoing, and I know I won't be alone."

"That is great to hear, Timmy. It really is rewarding for me to see people like you make the transformation with their lifestyles.

"Now that we had our break and are done with our snacks, let's get back to learning. We just discussed the importance of controlling insulin in the body and the roles that fats, carbs, and protein play. Now we are going to look at each macronutrient by itself so that you can learn a little bit more about each, but more importantly, what to eat."

"This is what I have been waiting for."

"I know it is. I have found that when you have a basic understanding of the 'why,' it makes doing it much easier."

"I agree. If you just told me to eat these things, I don't think it would have the same impact as you telling me how the body works and why I should eat them."

Matthew nodded at Timmy.

"Let's look at fats. Now you already know that fats don't have any effect on insulin secretion, but they do slow the absorption of carbohydrates into the system, which minimizes insulin spikes. Plus it…"

Timmy jumped in, "It also secretes a hormone that tells the brain to stop eating."

"Very good. You really like that point, don't you?"

Timmy smiled. "I just think it is really cool to learn how the body works. It just makes so much sense."

"Now I want to talk about the three types of fat: saturated, polyunsaturated, and monounsaturated."

"Is this going to get really scientific?"

"It can, but I am going to keep this simple for you.

"As a general rule, you want to avoid and minimize your intake of saturated fat. Excessive consumption of saturated fat can lead to diseases like heart disease, high cholesterol, and diabetes."

"Where do I find saturated fat? In what kinds of foods?"

"Glad you asked. I was going there next. Saturated fats are found primarily in animal proteins like liver, fatty red meats, and egg yolks.

"The fats that you want to consume are the unsaturated fats, these are either polyunsaturated or monounsaturated. As a general rule, these are your healthy fats. They can be found primarily in fish, nuts, and vegetable oils."

"Is there a fat that will help the body burn fat the best?"

"Great question, and actually there is. You want to make sure you are eating monounsaturated fats, those are the healthiest fats for the body and the ones that help you burn fat.

"There is something special about these fats as well."

"What's that?" asked Timmy as he cocked his head to the side.

"The healthy monounsaturated fats are some of the best tasting fats. They are found in foods like avocados, olives and olive oil, and in nuts like almonds, cashews, pistachios, and macadamia nuts.

"So not only are those fats tasty and healthy, they are also very easy to carry around."

Timmy nodded his head. "That is why you have almonds with a lot of your snacks. They provide you with healthy monounsaturated fats, they tell your brain to stop eating, and they slow the absorption of carbohydrates into the system."

"Give me a high five!" Matthew stood up and their hands collided together.

"This is really cool!" exclaimed Timmy.

"Yes it is. I know things can get a bit confusing with all of the fats out there, so I want to give you this other piece of information."

"What's that?"

"As a general rule, you want to stick with fats that are liquid at room temperature. These fats will be healthier for you."

"So that means that olive oil is healthier than butter or margarine because it is liquid and those are solid at room temperature?"

"You nailed it.

"Here are the foods that I generally eat to get my healthy fats. Some of my favorites are almonds, avocados, organic or natural peanut butter, olive oil and olive oil based salad dressings, lean meats, and assorted nuts like peanuts, pistachios, macadamia, and cashews."

"Why did you specifically say natural or organic peanut butter?"

"That is a great question, Timmy. The reason I said organic or natural peanut butter is because they do not have the hydrogenated oils added to them to make them creamy at room temperature. You should try to avoid hydrogenated oils as much as possible."

"What are hydrogenated oils?"

"They are very unhealthy fats that are used because they are cheap, and they keep products solid at room temperature."

"What do you mean?"

"Have you ever seen natural peanut butter, and how you will get a little bit of oil separation?"

"Of course I have."

"I know you have seen Jif or Skippy, and how creamy those peanut butters are at room temperature. I am sure you have also seen icing and frostings on cakes that don't need to be refrigerated."

"Definitely."

"Well, those products use hydrogenated oils. They are also found in shortenings and margarine."

"So basically, I should just avoid hydrogenated oils and trans fats."

"Exactly."

"Go ahead and write this down. Here are the basic guidelines that I follow for fat:

1. Eat fats that are liquid at room temperature. I use olive and canola oil.
2. Eat fish, raw nuts such as almonds / cashews / pistachios / macadamia / peanuts, and avocado.
3. Eat LESS corn, safflower, and sunflower oils.
4. And finally, eliminate hydrogenated oils and trans fats from your meals."

"That seems simple enough," said Timmy as he finished writing it all down. "I do have a few questions, though. You said egg yolks are high in saturated fats, and that they should be avoided."

"Yes. Egg yolks do have saturated fat, but they also have protein and other nutrients. It really comes down to the amount that you are eating. I stick to egg whites because of the amount of eggs I eat on a daily and weekly basis.

"Every now and then, it is ok to have egg yolks, but if you are eating eggs consistently, I would stick to just the egg whites."

"Sounds good. I will just follow your recommendation and stick to egg whites most of the time."

Timmy paused for a second to take in all that he has learned. "It is just hard to believe that for years 'no-fat' was all the rage." Then he chuckled, "My family was eating no-fat, but all we were getting was fat. Now it all makes sense. I am so glad you taught me this."

"You're welcome, Timmy. Your time will come as people will be looking to you for help in the near future. Then you will be able to turn around and be the teacher to somebody like yourself.

"Let's take a quick break and when we come back, we can learn about carbohydrates and protein."

"Sounds like a plan," said Timmy as he hopped up from his seat and headed down the hall.

29

Let's Talk About Carbs

"Let's keep the momentum going," said Timmy as he sat back down. "I already know that carbohydrates are what cause the body to secrete insulin, so now I'm ready for more information."

Matthew laughed. "Yes, now it's time to talk about the latest and greatest 'bad guy' on the block…carbohydrates!

"Just as you brought up before the break, for years our country went gaga over no-fat and low-fat, but then things changed. With the popularity of the Atkins diet and others that promoted a low- to no-carb regimen, carbohydrates replaced fats and became the new 'enemy.'"

Matthew did his best Hollywood sigh. "We just don't do moderation very well as a country."

Timmy nodded his head in agreement.

"You already mentioned there was a time when your family thought they could eat as much as they wanted of anything that was low- or no-fat."

"Yup."

"Well, the same thing happened with carbs. I knew things were out of hand when you started seeing double-bacon cheeseburgers with NO bun, being marketed to the 'no carb' dieters as being healthy."

"We would laugh at those people," said Timmy. "I remember being at a fast-food joint with my brother and watching people eat the same double-bacon cheeseburger I was eating, except instead of a bun, they had two pieces of lettuce. I just thought it was dumb."

Matthew just shook his head and smiled.

"That is the thing, Timmy, there was just so much misinformation about those low- and no-carb diets out there."

"You just said the word 'diet,'" he said as he pointed at Matthew with a sarcastic look of surprise on his face.

"I am glad that you noticed my use of the word 'diet' in there. I did that for a reason as you cannot go 'no carb' for very long and still function."

The smile faded from Timmy's face. "But wait a second; don't those low-carb diets work?

"The answer is YES, they DO work, but you have to be knowledgeable about them. Every bodybuilder or fitness model that is getting ready for a contest or photo shoot cuts carbs to prepare for the shoot or the competition."

"Really?"

"Yes, but they realize that it only provides short-term results for a contest or a photo shoot. That is why those diets got so popular so fast. People lost 'weight' pretty quickly when they started those diets.

"Why do you think that happened?"

"Let's see," said Timmy. "I would have to go back to our friend glycogen that you talked about a few weeks ago."

"What was glycogen again?" asked Matthew.

"It is the stored carbohydrates in the muscle and it acts like a sponge in that it holds water.

"That is also why people lose weight quickly, but it is mostly water weight. Since they aren't eating any carbs, doesn't that mean no insulin is produced, and therefore the body will burn fat?"

"Yes, the body will start to burn fat, but how long do you think you can go without carbs?"

"I don't know. I haven't tried it, but I'm guessing it isn't something you can do long-term"

"Not really. After a few days, you will feel tired, weak, and even light headed. You see, the body and the brain need carbohydrates."

"Have you ever done it, Matthew?"

"I have never done 'no-carb,' but I have done very low carb diets in the past when I had some photo shoots.

"I will tell you that it works, but only in the short term, and you can only really see the results once you are down well below 10% body fat."

"Wow, that is pretty low," said Timmy.

"Yup. I have seen people that were training for fitness contests almost pass out because they were so carb depleted.

"There is nothing wrong with bodybuilders or fitness professionals doing that to their bodies in the short term for a set purpose. But that is NOT what I teach people as it isn't the basis for a healthy lifestyle. I want to teach people habits they can use the rest of their life."

"That makes sense to me, but it is interesting to learn about these popular 'diets' that you hear about.

"I agree with you though Matthew, I like the idea of living a lifestyle so that I don't need crash diets."

"That is exactly it. If you keep doing what we are talking about, not only will you be very healthy, but also you will be able to enjoy food and eating. Trust me; once you get to your ideal weight, maintaining is a lot easier than having to lose weight."

"I am sure it is."

"That doesn't mean you can go back to your old habits; it just gives you more flexibility in that you don't have to be at a deficit every day to burn that extra fat."

"I understand," said Timmy.

"We got a little sidetracked on our discussion of no-carb diets, so back to the discussion of carbs."

"Hey Matthew, real fast, what carbs are the ones that we should be eating?"

"You read my mind. I was just about to go there.

"In an effort to keep things simple, you want to primarily eat naturally occurring carbs and minimize the consumption of junk carbs, which for simplicity sake we will call refined or processed carbohydrates."

"Matthew, I…"

"Let me finish, then I will answer your question."

"Healthy carbs are those carbs that are still in their natural state, meaning they haven't been processed or altered my humans.

These carbs are usually high in fiber and provide lasting energy to the body.

"Here are some examples of healthy carbohydrates:

- Fresh fruits & vegetables. Be aware that most canned fruits have lots of sugar added to make them even sweeter.
- Whole grain breads, pastas, crackers, and cereals. Again, these foods should still be eaten in moderation and in a meal complete with healthy fats and protein."

"Sounds simple enough. What I'm worried about are the 'bad carbs,' though. What are those?"

"The 'bad' carbs or the carbs you want to minimize on a day-to-day basis are the carbs that are refined or processed. These carbs are not in their natural state, which means they have to be processed. They are usually found in nice boxes or fancy packaging as opposed to growing on a tree or from the ground.

"A good rule of thumb is that junk carbs are usually very 'easy' to carry around and eat. A good example would be those 100-calorie snack packs. Sure, it is only 100 calories, but it is mostly refined and processed carbohydrates, with little to no fiber or protein.

"Here are some examples of your 'bad carbs':

- Most snack crackers
- Chips
- Cookies
- Sodas
- Cakes and brownies
- Candy bars
- 'Sugar' cereals. You know, the tasty ones that are more like dessert than a healthy way to start your day. They are super sweet, usually brightly colored, or actually have sugar sticking to the cereal."

"Wait a second," said Timmy. "You just said to avoid most snack crackers, yet we are eating Triscuits."

"Great point, Timmy. Triscuits are an example of a cracker that is good to eat."

"Can I substitute Wheat Thins for Triscuits since I like those as well?"

"You could, but I don't consider Wheat Thins to be in the same league as Triscuits."

"What do you mean?" asked Timmy.

"This is perfect timing because this leads into my next point. I just happen to have cut the sides off the boxes, so let's take a look at the ingredients contained in Triscuits and Wheat Thins."

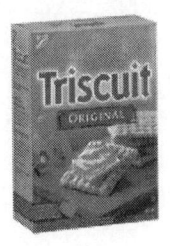

Ingredients: WHOLE WHEAT, SOYBEAN AND/OR PALM OIL, SALT.

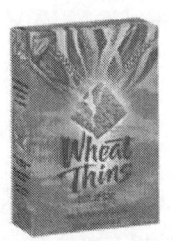

Ingredients: WHOLE GRAIN WHEAT FLOUR, UNBLEACHED ENRICHED FLOUR (WHEAT FLOUR, NIACIN, REDUCED IRON, THIAMINE MONONITRATE [VITAMIN B1], RIBOFLAVIN [VITAMIN B2], FOLIC ACID), SOYBEAN OIL, SUGAR, CORNSTARCH, MALT SYRUP (FROM BARLEY AND CORN), INVERT SUGAR, MONOGLYCERIDES, SALT, VEGETABLE COLOR (ANNATTO EXTRACT, TURMERIC OLEORESIN). CONTAINS: WHEAT. BHT ADDED TO PACKAGING MATERIAL TO PRESERVE FRESHNESS.

"Notice anything?" asked Matthew.

"Wait a second. Are you telling me that Triscuits have only three ingredients--whole wheat, oil, and salt--and that Wheat Thins have five or six *lines* of ingredients?"

"You nailed it."

"I can't even pronounce some of the stuff in Wheat Thins," said Timmy, shaking his head.

"Are Wheat Thins terrible for you? No, but the whole point of this is to illustrate what I am talking about with processed carbohydrates. The Triscuits are simple. Any third grader knows what those three ingredients are.

"This just reinforces what I am saying about eating carbs that are as natural as possible. That is why you want a bulk of your carbohydrates coming from fruits and veggies, and then making healthier decisions when you do grab crackers or other snack food. It is just about being aware."

"I get it. I guess we can apply your 'little things over time can make a big difference' to this as well, right?"

Matthew laughed. "We sure can. It isn't to say that you can't eat Wheat Thins every now and then, but if you consistently stick to choosing the more natural, less processed product, you will notice a difference in the long run."

"Let me guess, most of the stuff I used to eat when I would stop by the 7-11 for a snack was junk."

"I don't know exactly what you were eating, but knowing the content of most food carried in those stores, I would have to say yes. The shelves are typically lined with processed carbs that are tasty, but loaded with preservatives, food coloring, refined white flour, and corn syrups.

"It is these typical snack foods that are pretty much void of any nutritional value and are considered by many dieticians to be 'empty carbs.'"

"The funny thing, Matthew, is that I actually forgot how good healthy food can taste. I was really surprised how much I enjoyed the simple, yet healthy snacks you gave me last week."

"Stick with it another two to three weeks and you won't find yourself eating, much less craving, the junk food anymore. I used to eat all of those junk foods and I told myself it didn't matter because I was burning the calories, but after making the switch, I really could tell a huge difference," said Matthew. "Now that you have grasped the difference between good and bad carbs, there is one other important topic to discuss. That topic is the glycemic index."

"Are you going to get scientific on me again?"

"Just a little bit. Since you already know about insulin and how it impacts the body, this will be pretty easy for you.

"Remember how carbohydrates tell the body to secrete insulin?"

"Yes, I remember that."

"Well, not all carbohydrates have the same effect on the secretion of insulin. Some carbs have a slow impact on glycogen levels, while others have a rapid impact and can send levels skyrocketing. Basically, the glycemic index tells you how a carbohydrate impacts insulin levels."

"Sounds easy enough. Based on what I know already, I am guessing that I want to eat mostly carbs that have a slow impact on glycogen levels?"

"That is correct," said Matthew. "See, I told you this was easy.

"You mainly want to eat what are called low-glycemic carbohydrates. What makes it easy is that these carbs are generally the healthiest. These are your fruits and vegetables. These are the carbs that typically have lots of fiber and digest slowly into your system.

"Most of the 'bad carbs' like your sugars and processed carbohydrates tend to be fast acting, or high-glycemic carbs, and will spike your insulin levels, taking you out of the fat-burning zone and putting you in the fat-storing zone."

"Let me guess," said Timmy. "Not only do I want to eat low-glycemic carbs, but this is also the reason why you want me to eat fats and protein with every meal."

"Yes…"

"Let me finish," said Timmy. "Fat and protein help slow the breakdown of carbohydrates, plus the hormonal benefit that fat tells the brain to stop eating, and protein secretes a hormone glucagon that is basically the opposite of insulin."

"You are really blowing me away today," said Matthew as a big smile crossed his face. It was the same look of pride a teacher gets when they see a student making big progress.

"When you eat this way, you will be giving your body solid nutrition multiple times per day, while simultaneously keeping your insulin levels on an even keel.

"You won't have the insulin spikes and sugar highs followed by the dreaded post-sugar crash, but more importantly, you will keep your body in a fat-burning process as opposed to a fat-storing process."

"And I want to do everything possible to keep my body burning fat," exclaimed Timmy! Is there a place where I can find the glycemic index of foods?"

"There are plenty of places online, but for now, just keep it simple and stick to fruits and vegetables as a bulk of your carbohydrates. I was going to mention this earlier, but fiber doesn't have any effect on insulin either. So foods that are high in fiber are very good to eat as well."

"That is very good to know about fiber. Are you sure I don't need a chart?"

"Personally, I think it is overkill at this point. If you want to look up the glycemic index of your food, fine, but for our purposes, let's keep it **KISS**."

"*Keep It Super Simple*. I will never forget that."

"Just know this: your fruits and vegetables are generally low, and your starches like breads, pasta, and grains will generally be high."

"That is simple and helps a lot!"

"Again, I want to keep this simple. Don't worry too much if your favorite food is high glycemic. That is why you will always try to eat fats and protein with a meal so that you can minimize the insulin spike that would occur if you ate just a carbohydrate by itself."

"Is that why you told me to eat peanut butter or some almonds with my apple?"

"That is exactly right. We never want to eat just carbohydrates for a meal, even if they are low-glycemic or high in fiber. Apples just so happen to be low-glycemic to begin with, but adding some fat and protein with peanut butter makes it a more balanced 'meal.'"

"Are there any high-glycemic fruits that I should watch out for?"

"There are really only two. Again, they are very healthy, but if your goal is to lose body fat, then I would minimize eating them until you are closer to your goal weight."

"What are they?"

"They are bananas and raisins. The reason I mention this is because a lot of people like to 'grab a banana' as a snack. It is easy to carry around, it tastes good, and it is easy to eat.

"Bananas are great for potassium and this is very important if you are doing lots of endurance exercise, but if your primary goal is to burn fat, then I would choose another fruit. But if you do want that banana, make sure you consume some fats and protein with it to minimize the insulin spike."

"I get it. These are just finer points, to really dial things in."

"Exactly. I was almost hesitant to bring it up. If it comes down to eating a bag of potato chips or a banana, I would definitely want you to choose the banana."

Timmy laughed. "I get it."

"I am giving you more in-depth info because you have shown that you are committed to doing this. For a lot of people, I would keep it very simple, but I think you can handle this."

"On the card I am going to give you, I am going to list things in their order of importance. I do it this way so that people can slowly build as they are ready.

"Like the reason I didn't start you out eating six times per day on our first meeting, as you weren't ready yet. It will help as more and more people start looking to you for help."

"Looking to me for help?"

"Yes. I know you don't see it yet, but it will happen. It will probably start even sooner, but just wait a few months. People will notice that you have lost a lot of weight and will want to talk to you about how you did it."

"Ahh, I see. So you are telling me people are going to start looking to me to answer their questions?"

"Why wouldn't they? They will have seen your body transform before their eyes over a semester or two. You will be somebody 'familiar' to them, and they will start to ask you questions."

"Ok, if you say so," replied Timmy, not convinced that anybody would ask him for help.

Matthew just nodded and smiled.

"I know we got a bit sidetracked there at the end of our discussion about carbohydrates, but let's take a short break and learn about protein."

"Perfect, my bladder is about to explode anyway," said Timmy as he popped out of his seat and hurried down the hall.

30

Let's Talk About Protein

Timmy burst into the office, slammed his fist on the desk, and in his best pro wrestler voice said, "Let's talk about some protein!"

Matthew laughed hysterically. "You're a piece of work, you know that?"

Timmy sat back down, grabbed his notebook, looked up at Matthew and said, "I'm ready to learn, if you're ready to teach." Then he burst out laughing.

"Do you know what I'm seeing with you?"

Timmy got serious for a second. "What?"

"I am seeing your personality come through. I am getting a glimpse of the real Timmy; not the one that is shy and thinks that everybody is talking about his weight. I am seeing the fun, outgoing, and humorous person that I don't think has come out for a long time."

Timmy just sat there, his eyes looking at the floor. "I don't know how to explain it, Matthew. I just feel as if the weight of the world has been lifted off my shoulders. I now realize that I don't have to be trapped in my body as it is now for the rest of my life. It is like I see a new beginning for me."

Matthew smiled and put his hand on Timmy's shoulder. "I completely understand. You have no idea the amazing things life has in store for you. Just keep doing what you are doing and keep your positive mental attitude and you will go far."

Timmy smiled and nodded. "Thanks Matthew. I see that you saved protein for last, is that because it is the best?"

Matthew chuckled. "No one nutrient is the best, as they all need each other. Protein is very important, as the body requires it to maintain and repair all of the muscles and cells in the body. Every process in the body needs and depends on protein, so yes, it is very important."

"I thought protein just built muscles?"

"It does do that, but it does so much more. On a scientific level, every enzyme in the body is made of protein, and these enzymes control all of the chemical reactions in the body."

"Wow, so protein is for more than just big muscles."

"Yes, Timmy, much more. In fact, when you talk to your sister and your mother, you should let them know the importance of protein. The reason I single them out is because generally I have found that most women don't get enough protein."

"Why should they care?" asked Timmy.

"Because protein is responsible for the overall maintenance and repair of the body. If they want to keep that radiant skin, healthy hair, and strong nails, and keep those bones strong later in life, you need to make sure they are getting enough protein."

Timmy nodded. "That makes sense. They spend a fortune on hair and beauty products, so I'm sure that will interest them."

"Good. Now let's take a closer look at protein.

"When you consume and digest protein, the protein is broken down into amino acids, which are then used to build and repair the body. There are twenty amino acids broken down into two main types, essential and non-essential.

"Essential amino acids are just that, essential! These amino acids are essential because they cannot be produced by the human body and must be consumed through food."

"Wait a second. So you are telling me that the body can produce certain amino acids?"

"Yes, the body can produce non-essential amino acids if they are not consumed in sufficient quantity through food, and as long as there are enough raw materials present in the liver to produce them.

"The goal is to consume enough complete protein, which contains all of the amino acids, so that our bodies don't have to produce their own. Incomplete proteins don't contain all the amino acids, but it is nice to know our bodies can produce these non-essential amino acids in case we come up short nutritionally."

Timmy smiled, nodded, and jotted a few things down in his notebook.

"There are two main sources of protein: plant and animal protein. Beans, nuts, and soy are good examples of plant protein. Some good sources of animal protein are chicken, beef, tuna, and eggs.

"It doesn't sound like you or anybody else in your family is a vegetarian, but it is important to note that most plant proteins are incomplete proteins. Aside from soy and a few other plant proteins, only animal proteins are complete proteins and supply all of the essential amino acids in the proper quantities that are necessary for the body."

"I got it. Try to eat complete proteins, and most plant proteins are not complete."

"That is good, but I don't want you to think that plant proteins are bad. You just might have to combine several plant proteins to get a complete protein. The other main reason animal protein is preferred by many over plant protein comes down to density."

"Density?"

"Yup. Some plant proteins contain a higher percentage of protein than many meats."

"Yeah, so what's wrong with that?"

"Nothing, the only issue is the density of the plant proteins. Whereas a half-pound of meat might only be the size of your fist, a half-pound of spinach could easily take 2-3 large plates to fill. Which one would you rather eat?"

Timmy laughed. "I get it. Most meats are dense, whereas most plant proteins are not. So you have to eat a lot more plant matter to get the same amount of protein as a much smaller piece of meat."

"Bingo. You got it."

"Ok then, so now that I understand how important protein is to the body, how much should I eat per day?"

"That is a great question and one that can have a very long and complex answer. I am going to do my best to keep this simple."

Timmy laughs. "Like you would have it any other way."

"The first thing we need to do is find out about what our lean body mass is. This is the weight of your body, minus the body fat.

"This can be done if you know your body fat percentage. I am going to assume that you, like most people, do not and do not have the ability to get it done easily. Plus, the more overweight a person is, the less reliable the easy methods like caliper tests are."

"So what is the best way to find out your lean body mass?"

"The most accurate way is called hydrostatic testing. That is where they weigh your entire body in and out of water with a special scale."

"Oh, I see. Sounds complicated."

"It can be, so this is what I want you to do. I want you to take your goal weight, which should be very close to the ideal weight for somebody your height anyway. Since you said you wanted to get down to 180, we will use that number.

"Once you find your ideal or goal weight, I want you to subtract 15% from that number, and if you share this information with your mom or sister, have them take off 25%."

"Why the difference?"

"The difference is that healthy women will naturally have about 10% higher body fat than men.

"So grab your calculator. Let's take your goal of 180 pounds, multiply by .15, which means that there is 27 pounds of body fat at normal levels. Subtract 27 from 180, and you get a target lean mass of 153 pounds."

"Wait a second; why not just use my body weight, or my ideal body weight?"

"Great question, Timmy. The reason is that body fat doesn't need protein to maintain itself. Only your lean body mass needs and uses protein for repair and maintenance."

"I get it. That makes a lot of sense. That way I am only consuming what my body needs, and not a lot of extra."

"Exactly. If you were a 300 pound bodybuilder, things would be different as you would have a much higher lean mass and very little body fat.

"Now that we know our lean mass, we want to aim to get 0.7 to 1.0 grams of protein per pound of lean body weight. If you aren't very active, shoot for the lower end, and if you are exercising several times per week, shoot for the higher range.

"What that means is that if you aren't very active, you need a minimum of about 107 grams of protein per day, and if you are pretty active, you need about 150 grams per day. Again, this is just a rough guide. It will not make or break you, but it will be better than not having a plan at all."

"That seems like a lot," said Timmy, as he continued to take notes.

"I am sure it does at first glance, but don't forget that we are spreading this out over five or six meals. Get fifteen to thirty grams of protein per meal, and you will easily hit those numbers.

"Again, I want to drive the point home that this is just a guide. If you really want to get it exact, it can be done, but it just takes some time, money, and effort. That said, let's do a hypothetical example for your sister."

"That is a great idea. She is overweight, just not near as bad as I am. I think I have heard her say she wants to lose like 30 pounds and get down to 140."

"Perfect, let's start there. To find her lean body mass, take the 140 pounds that she wants to be and multiply .25, which gives us 35 pounds of fat. Subtract that from 140, which gives us a lean mass of 105 pounds. She is going to need anywhere from about 73 to 105 grams of protein per day."

"That is actually pretty easy."

"I am glad you think so. I think it is a good balance between being easy and being fairly accurate. The goal is to get people headed in the right direction. Once they start heading that way, they usually take it upon themselves to dial things in if that is what they want. Most will be happy with a good guide and the results it produces."

"I agree with you on that. I want to take things to the next level, but I also see how a lot of people would be happy with good results. That said, how much protein do you aim for each day, Matthew?"

"Personally, I aim towards the higher end of the spectrum. Since I have a background of working out very hard, and my body fat is in the single digits, I typically shoot for a minimum of one gram per pound of lean body mass. This has been my guide for over twenty years and works very well for me."

"Wow that is pretty cool that you have been able to do that for twenty years."

"I know it seems hard at first, but trust me, it will become a part of your lifestyle and is actually pretty easy to do.

"Now that we know how much protein we should be aiming for each day, let's figure out the best way to consume that amount.

"The best sources of protein are chicken, turkey, tuna, lean meats, eggs, milk, nuts, and soy."

"What makes one protein better than another?"

"There are several things, but I don't want to get too complicated. For our purposes, we want to consume lean proteins, meaning proteins that do not have a lot of saturated fat. I also like to get a lot of my protein from complete proteins, that way I know my body has enough amino acids to repair itself.

"I am glad you asked that question as I do have a quick tip that I want to share with you. When choosing an animal protein, the fewer legs the better."

Timmy shook his head. "What?"

Matthew chuckled. "If you have a choice between pork and chicken for your protein, choose chicken. Two legs versus four."

Timmy laughed. "I get it now. I was just spacing out for a second."

"No problem. This is just a simple rule as chicken and fish tend to be leaner than protein from our four legged friends such as beef or pork."

"I know you touched on it earlier, so I figured I would ask about it now."

"What's that?" enquired Matthew.

"Protein shakes."

"Ah yes, protein shakes. I bet I know what you are thinking. Those are only for muscle head guys; they taste like chalk and water, and there is no way I'm ever going to do that."

"Sort of, but since everything else you have told me seems to work, why wouldn't I trust you on protein shakes as well? I guess it will just take some getting used to."

"I understand where you are coming from. Trust me; you aren't the first person to be turned off by hearing about protein shakes. The thing is, protein is so important to the body, and it's one of the nutrients that I believe most people, especially women, don't get enough of.

"As somebody who has taken various protein supplements since I was a young kid, I can tell you that things have come a long way. Not just in the quality of the protein, but more importantly in the taste!

"What if I told you that I had a protein powder that mixed instantly with water and had no chunks or chalky texture? Would you look at trying it?"

"I guess. Never hurts to try," responded Timmy.

"Good. My personal favorite flavor tastes like a less intense Hawaiian Punch or berry flavored drink, and it is the flavor that I recommend to my friends and to their wives and girlfriends."

"Wait a second, you recommend protein shakes to women? And they actually try them?"

"You bet they do. Once they learn the value of consuming enough protein--meaning healthy hair, skin, and nails--it really helps get them on board. Then once they taste it, they are usually sold on the idea."

"Really?"

"Really. Just so happens I made you a little sample for today."

Matthew pulled out a water bottle that had a reddish pink liquid inside.

"This is the berry flavored protein I was telling you about. Here, try it."

Timmy reached for the water bottle, unscrewed the top, and sniffed it as if he was expecting to be repulsed.

He put the bottle to his lips and took a sip.

"Hey, that is actually pretty good. And you're telling me that is healthy? Cool!"

"I am glad you find it tolerable," said Matthew with a laugh. "I want to walk you through something, so just bear with me, ok?"

"Sure, what is it?"

"Let's look at this for a second. How long would it take you to eat an entire chicken breast?"

"I don't know, seven to fifteen minutes sounds reasonable."

"Perfect," said Matthew. "How long would it take you to prepare this chicken?"

"Let's see, anywhere from twelve to forty minutes, depending on if you grill it or bake it."

"Sounds about right."

"Um, where are you going with this, Matthew?"

"What if I told you that one scoop of that great tasting protein powder could be mixed in eight to ten ounces of water and have just as much, if not more, high quality protein than an entire chicken breast or piece of steak?"

"Really?"

"Yes, and how long do you think it would take you to drink eight to ten ounces of water?"

"I could chug it in less than ten seconds, but if I were just going to drink it, I don't know, I will say two to five minutes for the sake of this example."

"Sounds very reasonable. How long would it take you to pour one scoop of powder into a glass or bottle and stir or shake it?"

"I would say fifteen seconds to a minute sounds reasonable. But where are you going with this?"

"Stay with me now. I am sure that you, along with pretty much every person I know, has complained at one point or another in their lives that they were too busy or didn't have enough time."

Timmy huffed. "Well sure, I think everybody has said that at one point or another in their lives, at least once."

"I know, Timmy. That was the point. Everybody wishes they had more time at some point or another."

"So what is your point though?"

"My point is that you can spend two to five minutes to prepare and consume the same amount of quality protein through a protein shake that would take twenty minutes to an hour to prepare and eat if it were real food."

"Oh, I get it now!" exclaimed Timmy.

"I am not telling you to stop eating real food by any means, but when you are going to be eating six times per day, quality protein is usually the toughest thing to get. Aside from nuts, protein isn't very easy to carry around unless you are using protein bars or shakes."

"That really makes it easy. You are right again, Matthew. I was worried about having to carry around ice packs for my cottage cheese and yogurt on certain afternoons, but now I know that I can put some protein powder in my water bottle and still be fine."

"Exactly. Fat and carbohydrates are 'easy' to eat and carry around. Protein takes a little planning and effort. That is why I want to make it easy for you! I don't want you to be afraid that protein powders or bars are just for bodybuilders."

Timmy laughed. "I am ready to try protein powder. I have to admit, I ate everything you gave me last week except for the protein powder. Is that the same powder you used to make the drink you just gave me?"

"It is exactly the same stuff. That said, I think it is time I let you in on a little secret."

Timmy perked up. "What's that Matthew?"

"Pretty much every guy or girl you see that has a lean and sexy body is taking some sort of protein supplement to complement his or her nutritional program."

"Really?"

"I wouldn't lie to you. Most of your top athletes and fitness and bikini models you see on TV and in the magazines and even Hollywood celebrities that need to get in shape for a role have taken some sort of protein supplement.

"There is no 'easy' way to a lean body other than through your nutrition program. When you eat protein, not only does it help repair your body so you create more lean mass, but the body burns calories just digesting and breaking down protein.

"And guess what happens when you get more lean mass?"

"Um, I'm not exactly sure."

"When you get more lean mass, your body burns more calories at rest. This means that your body burns more calories when it is doing nothing as lean mass raises your metabolism."

"I like that. Burning more calories at rest can only help the weight come off."

"You are correct.

"I do want to bring this up in case you talk with your mom, sister, or other women about protein shakes down the road. I know that many women feel that if they take protein shakes or start working out that they will somehow start looking like the women bodybuilders.

"Nothing could be farther from the truth. All they will do is end up doing is being toned and healthy. The guys are trying to put on muscle as fast as they can. They are working out, eating protein, and will try anything under the sun in the hopes of putting on muscle fast, and it still doesn't happen quickly. It takes time."

"Makes sense. I will be sure to tell Jessica not to worry about looking like a bodybuilder," said Timmy sarcastically.

Matthew just shook his head and smirked.

"Now that we have covered the basics with fats, carbohydrates, and protein, I just need to teach you how to read food labels, as well as touch on two more important aspects of your nutritional program: water and vitamins."

"Sounds like a plan," said Timmy. "Let's take a break and knock the rest of this out today!"

"I like your enthusiasm. See you back here in five minutes."

Matthew and Timmy left the office to start their break.

31

Putting It All Together – How to Build Your Meals

"Ok, Matthew. I'm ready to rock. You have taught me a lot the past few weeks. I know that I need to eat five to six times per day. I know that I need to eat fat, carbs, and protein at each meal. But how do I put all of this together?"

"I like your excitement. That is what we are going to discuss right now. Before I get into this, I want to make a few things perfectly clear."

Timmy nodded his head.

"First, one thing I see happen with a lot of people is that they get overwhelmed. They start reading too much or trying to make things so much harder than it really is. Remember, it is just food.

"Second, if you eat too much or have a bad meal, just put it behind you. If you have a few bad meals in a row, same thing--put it behind you and get back on track. Here is one thing I like to tell people: You can't get fat in day, and you can't get skinny in a day either."

"Matthew, it seems like you are worried that you are giving me too much detail and information."

"I am worried a little bit. No matter what it is, when things get hard or complex, you lose people. They end up thinking that the only way to get results is to do these complex things, and that just isn't the case. I want to make it easy to understand and I want most people to see a healthy lifestyle as a realistic opportunity for themselves."

"I hear you, Matthew. I didn't know squat about eating healthy, but now I feel like I have a really good understanding. I know things are very complex, but I also think you did an amazing job at making it easy to understand. After a few semesters of health and biology classes, I never understood this much about the body until I started working with you."

"Thanks, Timmy. I appreciate that. Everybody learns in different ways, so I want to be effective and reach as many people as possible, and I don't want to turn people off or scare them away. Being healthy is really pretty easy, and I think most health and fitness people, myself included, can get a little too into the weeds."

"I understand, but remember, I asked for you to take things to the next level."

"Yes you did, and that is why I have put together a great little handout that gives you the steps you can take when you are ready."

"Awesome! I can't wait to see it."

"Well, here it is. Let me know what you think."

Timmy took the sheet of paper, momentarily flipping it back and forth to see that there was writing on both sides.

"I have a quick question."

"Sure, what is it?"

"Is this a KISS handout?"

Matthew laughed.

"Yes, it is definitely KISS. Don't worry about calories, hormones, insulin, or enzymes; just follow the easy guidelines below and you will be just fine."

Timmy smiled. "I like that a lot."

"Great, now take a minute or two to read that sheet so you can let me know what you think."

"Ok."

32

The Lean Life "KISS" Handout

Level 1 – The Basics – Do these 4 things over time & you will be in shape!

1. **Just Move!** Walk, walk, and walk some more. It doesn't have to be scheduled, but just make a point to walk more during the day. Park farther away, take more breaks at work, walk after lunch, etc.
2. **Drink water!** It doesn't get much simpler than that. Your body is 70% water, and you need more water if you want to burn body fat. Add lemon or cucumber for flavor. Swapping just ONE soda or fruit juice for water each day will save you 15 pounds over the course of a year! Shoot for 8 glasses to a gallon per day.
3. **Small plates!** Portion control is key. Eat your meals on salad plates, and use small bowls for cereals, soups, and desserts. Trick your mind. A 'full' small plate looks better than the same food on a large plate with empty space.
4. **Posture!** Do the Lean Life Squeeze. Feet straight ahead, tighten your glutes (butt muscles), then your abs, and then pull your shoulders back, and stand tall with your head high. Hold it for 10 seconds to a minute or longer. Do it anytime anywhere. Nobody has to know!

Level 2 – The Next Steps – For those that want to get there faster.

- Eat 5 to 6 times per day. Have your 3 regular meals, and add a 'mini-meal' (snack) between lunch & dinner and before bed. If you eat breakfast more than 5 hours before you eat lunch, eat a mini-meal mid-morning. Mini-meals should be about ½ to ¾ the size of the palm of your hand.
- Each meal should contain fats, carbohydrates, and protein. You want to avoid eating 'just carbohydrates' for any snack or meal.

Level 3 – Dial it in! - You are ready to maximize your fat loss and get in top shape! Build Your Meals - note: mini-meals should be about 1/3 the size of your meals

Step 1 – Choose a lean protein that is about the size of the palm of your hand.

Chicken, tuna, turkey, egg whites, low-fat cottage cheese, low-fat Greek yogurt, soy, or lean red meat are good examples.

Step 2 – Add carbohydrates, preferably in the form of fruits and vegetables. If adding fruits and veggies, which are generally "low-glycemic," add DOUBLE the size of your protein portion. If you are adding rice, grains, bread, or pasta, which are generally high-glycemic, make it the SAME size as the protein portion. Here are two simple guidelines; the rest is up to you!

- Fruits & veggies - most are great, so eat up! Minimize: bananas, raisins.
- Best grains to eat – oatmeal, beans. Minimize most grains, bread, and pasta.

Step 3 – Add healthy fats that are about the size of your thumb. You want to consume poly & mono *unsaturated* fats, minimize saturated fats, and avoid all trans fats and hydrogenated oils.

- Best choices: almonds, avocado, olive oil, canola oil, natural peanut butter, cashews, macadamia nuts, peanuts, and omega-3 fish oil.
- Avoid/minimize: fatty red meats, egg yolks, organ meats like liver, shortenings, sour cream, cream cheese, cream, and butter.

Step 4 – Time to eat! Start by eating your fats and protein. Fats will signal the brain to "stop eating" as well as slow the digestion of carbohydrates and release of insulin into the system. Protein triggers hormones that counteract the insulin release from the carbohydrates. That is why you want fat and protein to reach your stomach first.

This is the natural way to keep your body burning fat while minimizing and eliminating cravings and the feeling that you need to keep eating. Let your body do the work naturally and you won't need to rely on willpower to stop eating.

Tips, Tricks, and Helpful Hints

- Drink a glass of water 20-30 minutes before every meal. Water helps you burn fat and will naturally make you feel full so you will eat less.
- This is easy; don't make it harder than it has to be. This is a guide you can loosely follow your entire life and still get great results. Always fall back on the basics: walk, water, and portion control!
- Share with others in your community. When you involve the people in your life, it makes the process easier because your family, friends, and co-workers work together with you towards the common goal of health. More info at: http://FitLife212.com

"Little things over time make a BIG difference!"

"I really like that a lot," said Timmy.

"Good, I am going to put together another one for you with a list of foods as well as some example snacks and meals."

"Awesome!"

"Do you know what is really cool?"

"No, what?"

"How would you like a little card you could print off and keep in your wallet that had the key points to help you when you were out and about?"

"That would be really nice. Not only is the information good, but every time I would open my wallet it would help keep me on track."

"My thoughts exactly," said Matthew. "I used to do a similar thing a while back. I had a card with motivational quotes on it that sat in my wallet. It helped my mindset every time opened my wallet to purchase something."

"That is a great idea. On our next break, can I go make some copies of this sheet?"

"Sure. Actually, why don't we take a break now? I need to grab some water and you can take that down to Sandy, John's assistant, and she can help you make the copies."

"Perfect. See you back here in just a few."

33

The Lean Life "KISS" Handout

"Get your copies?"

"Yes, I got them. You know Matthew, Sandy is really nice."

"I know; she is great."

"It wasn't just that she stopped what she was doing to help me with the copies, but she said the nicest thing to me."

"What did she say?"

"She said that she has seen me coming in here every week to meet with you and John and that she can see the results already. Not just in my weight, but in how I carry myself. She also smiled and told me to keep up the great work."

"See, I told you it was about way more than just weight. It is going to take time for you to lose your weight, but you can change your mindset and how you present yourself almost overnight. You just had to start believing in yourself."

"I know. It is still something I have to fight every day."

"I understand completely. You might find this hard to believe, but I used to have a hard time believing in myself too."

"You? Sorry Matthew, but I'm not buying it."

"It is true. I had real issues with being perfect. It started when I was young, and I felt that I had to be perfect."

"What do you mean by 'perfect?'" asked Timmy with a puzzled look on his face.

"Exactly, what does it mean? That was the problem, I was trying to live up to some standard I thought was being placed on me by somebody else, but actually it was my incorrect interpretation of things as a kid. That stuck with me for many years."

"Really? I just assumed you had some perfect life."

"See, we throw around this word 'perfect,' but what does it mean? Perfect job, perfect body, perfect husband or perfect wife?"

"I see what you mean," said Timmy.

"Yes, I learned that things, and specifically myself, would never be perfect. Once I got over that mental block that had been holding me back for years, I too began to change the way I carried myself."

Timmy smiled and nodded. "It is pretty cool that you shared that with me, Matthew. It makes sense though."

"So even though I was never fighting a 'weight' battle, I know what it feels like when your own mind is keeping you down. Like you, I had to fight it all the time for a while. It was a constant battle because you are getting there, but you don't quite believe it yet.

"Same thing with your weight, you are getting there, but you still don't quite believe it yet. I know it is going to be a battle that you are going to have to fight for a while. At some point, I have a friend out in San Diego that I want you to talk with."

"Ok. Why is that?"

"Well, she is a friend of mine that used to be obese. She was about ten pounds heavier than you, but she was only five feet three inches tall."

"Really? My weight?"

"Yes, your weight."

"How is she doing now?"

"She is doing great. She lost 167 pounds."

"Whoa! That is awesome!"

"Yes, it is awesome. She was an inspiration to me. I learned so much from talking with her. So even though I haven't had to fight weight, she gave me a glimpse of what goes on inside the head of somebody that is. Meeting her gave me a newfound compassion for people in general."

"I can see that," replied Timmy. "I hope that I can talk to her at some point."

"I will see what I can do. That said, are you ready to learn how to read food labels?"

"You bet I am!"

"We are going to start with this label that I pulled off a box of crackers."

Matthew handed Timmy a sheet of paper with a photocopy of the label.

"I made a photocopy of the label and I figured it would be easier to take notes this way."

Nutrition Facts
Serving Size 5 Crackers (16g)
Servings Per Container About 28

Amount Per Serving	
Calories 80	Calories from Fat 40

	% Daily Value*
Total Fat 4.5g	**7%**
Saturated Fat 1g	5%
Trans Fat 0g	
Polyunsaturated Fat 1.5g	
Monounsaturated Fat 2g	
Cholesterol 0mg	**0%**
Sodium 140mg	**6%**
Total Carbohydrate 9g	**3%**
Dietary Fiber less than 1g	1%
Sugars 1g	
Protein 1g	

Vitamin A 0%	•	Vitamin C 0%
Calcium 0%	•	Iron 2%

*Percent Daily Values are based on a 2,000 calorie diet. Your daily values may be higher or lower depending on your calorie needs:

		Calories	2,000	2,500
Total Fat	Less than		65g	80g
Sat Fat	Less than		20g	25g
Cholesterol	Less than		300mg	300mg
Sodium	Less than		2,400mg	2,400mg
Total Carbohydrate			300g	375g
Dietary Fiber			25g	30g

"The first thing I want you to do when looking at a label is give the label a quick scan. Start at the top with the serving size and servings per container.

"This is especially important with processed foods and 'dessert' type foods as companies will try to make them appear to be lower in calories and fat by adjusting the serving size."

"What do you mean?"

"They will 'shrink' the serving size to make the calories and fat look like it is less. You will see a small box or jar of a product and it says 'only 90 calories per serving' on the box."

"That doesn't sound like a lot."

"It might not be, but you have to look at the servings per container to see what that means. If you have two equal size products, both with 90 calories per serving, but product A has five servings in the box and product B has thirty servings per box, which one do you think you can eat more of?"

"Oh I see. If you got out of control and ate the entire box of product A, that would only be 450 calories, but if you ate the entire box of product B, that would be like 2700 calories."

"Exactly! So always look at the serving size and the servings per container. In the example above, the serving size is five crackers and there are twenty-eight servings in the box. Now, those could be very small crackers, or they could be big crackers, but at least you have a good idea as to the serving size."

"I understand. What's next?"

"Work your way down the label. Check out the calories and notice the calories from fat. It says forty calories from fat. How many calories in a gram of fat, Timmy?"

"That's too easy, Matthew. There are nine."

Matthew gave Timmy a sly smile. "Good to see that you're paying attention.

"So we then move down to see there are 4.5 grams of fat in the crackers. Since we know there are 9 calories per gram, 4.5 multiplied by 9 is about 40, so the label is accurate.

"Now we want to look at the breakdown of the fat. It has most of the fat coming from the healthy unsaturated fats, and only 1 gram of saturated fat. It also has zero trans fats, which is great. If you see trans fats, put the product back on the shelf as there are probably better alternatives.

"So all in all, as far as fats go, these crackers have a pretty good fat content."

"Even with the saturated fat?"

"Yes. One gram of saturated fat isn't very much. You can see out to the side that it is only five percent of the recommended daily value for saturated fat. Again, moderation is key. Half of the fat is from monounsaturated fats, which is great, and another thirty percent is polyunsaturated fat. With eighty percent being healthy fat, you have nothing more to worry about here.

"Next, we keep moving down to look at the cholesterol and sodium. Just look to the side where it says '% daily value' and see if there are high percentages there. Cholesterol can clog your arteries, and sodium is another word for salt. If you are healthy, just keep an eye on those categories, but for people with high blood pressure, these two lines are very important."

Timmy nodded as he continued to take notes.

"Next we want to look at the total carbohydrates. These crackers have nine grams total, with less than one gram of fiber, and only one gram of sugar. Since these are crackers, they are probably made from refined grains. These grains don't offer much fiber or sugar, but they are just insulin-producing carbs."

"Isn't it good that they are low in sugar?"

"It could be, but sugar isn't the enemy. If you look at a piece of fruit like an apple, or skim milk, you will see that ALL of the carbs come from sugar. The natural sugar in apples and milk are generally better for you than the processed carbohydrates from grains and crackers.

"Then we come to protein. Protein is important because it is the key macronutrient we are going to base our meals around. We need to make sure we are getting those fifteen to thirty-five grams per meal."

"So what do we do since this product only has one gram of protein?"

"Good question, what do you think we should do?"

"I don't know," replied Timmy.

"What did we do with the Triscuits I gave you last week?"

"You put peanut butter on them."

"Exactly, but does that mean peanut butter is the only thing I could put on these?"

"No, but what else could you do?" inquired Timmy.

"I could put little pieces of lean turkey or low-fat cottage cheese on these crackers. I could even eat these crackers by themselves, but mix a half scoop of protein powder in water to drink with it."

Timmy's face lit up. "I get it; you can use food to build whatever it is that you need."

"Exactly. Let's say I have some fat-free yogurt that only has carbs and protein, what could I do?"

"You could eat some almonds with it, you could mix some nuts in with the yogurt, or you could mix some peanut butter in as well," said Timmy.

"That was pretty easy, wasn't it?"

"What if you were eating something that had mostly fat and protein, but no carbohydrates? What would you do then?"

"Depending on what it was, I would try to add either fruits or vegetables to complete the meal."

"Are there any things alone that can be good snacks?"

"There are, but most things are going to require a little combining of some sort. Take low-fat Greek yogurt for example. It has a healthy amount of fat, a lot of protein, but lacking on carbs. So what could we do?"

Timmy thought to himself but looked puzzled. "Oh wait, I get it! I could just add some fruit to the yogurt. I could add blueberries, strawberries, apple pieces, or all of the above."

Matthew smiled as he sat back in his chair. He didn't have to say anything this time, Timmy just looked at him, and the expression on Matthew's face told him everything he needed to know. His mentor was proud of him.

"I do have a question though. Since we didn't really talk about calories and grams of fat, protein, carbs, do you have any guidelines?"

"Sure I do, but just in case, you can always visualize the portion sizes. Since a piece of lean protein the size of the palm of your hand will have about twenty-five grams of protein, that will be our starting point. What comes next after the protein?"

Timmy quickly checked his notes. "Carbohydrates. If they are fruits or veggies, they can be twice the size; if grains, pasta, or bread, it can be the same size."

"Exactly right. An apple will have about twenty grams of carbohydrates, and two apples are about double the size of your palm, so that would be forty grams of carbs. Ideally, that is what we want to shoot for. Anything from thirty to forty-five grams of carbohydrates would be fine."

"So let me guess, since we visualize a sliver on the plate the size of my thumb, I am going to guess that is going to be about eight to ten grams of fat."

"Exactly. Assuming there isn't much fat in the meal already, you will want to eat almonds, olive oil, avocado, or other nuts to get that eight to ten grams of fat. Assuming there is a lot of fat already in the meal, you might not have to add any fat."

"Whew," Timmy sighed. "I actually think I have a good grasp on this."

"I believe that you do. I told you it wasn't that complicated."

Timmy laughed. "Yeah right, you were the one all worried that you were making it too complicated."

"Well, I'm glad you get it and understand it. That is what counts."

"Is there anything else I need to know or look out for?"

"There are a few things. You see the '% daily value?'"

"Yes, I see it."

"Those percentages are based on a 2000 calorie per day diet. If you were an athlete that needs 6000 calories per day, you could divide the percentage listed by 3. Conversely, if you were on a 1000-calorie per day diet, you would need to double those percentages listed. Does that make sense?"

"I get the second part, but not the first."

"Ok. Let's say that the food gives you 15% of the recommended sodium intake for the day. Since you need to eat 3x the 2000 calorie diet, that 15% would need to be divided by 3, as that same amount of food on a 6000 calorie diet is only 5%."

"I got it. I don't know why I didn't see that."

"The only other thing to touch on is to look at the ingredients. Like we discussed earlier, try to choose foods with fewer ingredients, or at least ingredients that recognize. If you can't pronounce half of the ingredients in the food, it might be better to grab something natural like an apple, skim milk, or nuts, as those will be healthier choices."

"That makes sense. It is so true what you said, once I started eating smaller portions and eating healthier food, I don't miss the stuff I used to eat very much at all."

Matthew nodded his head in agreement. "It usually takes two to four weeks to create a new habit. Some are easier than others. I am glad that you are enjoying your new eating habits. These habits will serve you well for the rest of your life.

"Anything else you can think of?"

"Yes, what are your thoughts on vitamins? Should I take them, and if so, which ones?"

RING…RING…RING

"Sorry Timmy, I have to grab this call. Why don't you take a quick break and we will pick back up in a minute."

"Sounds good, Matthew."

Timmy left the office while Matthew took his phone call.

34

Vitamins

"I apologize, Timmy, but I had to take that call."

"It's fine. I needed a break anyway."

"So what was your question before we were interrupted?"

"I wanted to know if I should be taking vitamins, and if so, which ones?"

"Here is the deal; vitamins can be a very touchy subject with some people. I will give you my opinion, and you can do as you see fit.

"First off, vitamins don't provide you with any energy. Only fats, carbs, and protein can do that. Sure, vitamins help with the many processes that go on in the body and they are a necessity, but you will get plenty of vitamins through the food that you eat, especially the way I have taught you."

"So what do you take?"

"I take a multi-vitamin, B-vitamin, and calcium; that's it."

"That's it?"

"As far as vitamins go, yes. I also take fish oil, which provides healthy omega-3 fats."

"I have seen people that get expensive vitamins, and I have seen them cheap at the drugstore. Which do you suggest?"

"I am not here to tell you what to do. As somebody who has tried and or been pitched pretty much every nutritional vitamin or supplement under the sun, here is my take--don't spend a lot of money on vitamins. I get all of my vitamins in bulk where I get 300-

500 tabs of each vitamin for around ten to fifteen bucks each. I spend about $45 and get a year's worth of vitamins.

"I have seen and tried vitamins that cost over $100 per month. Did I feel a difference? Not really. But I will admit, the packaging was cool, and the salespeople really believed in those vitamins."

Timmy laughed.

"I started taking vitamins while I was still in diapers, and have for the past thirty plus years. When I was competing with top swim programs, they gave us vitamins. Do you think they gave us fancy-dancy expensive vitamins?"

"I'm going to guess, no."

"You would be correct.

"That said, I know you will run into people that are taking expensive vitamins and they will swear they are the best thing since the Internet. They will tell you about absorption and a whole host of other stuff. I just nod and smile. I am comfortable with my cheap vitamins and healthy food; it works for me, just as their expensive vitamins work for them."

Timmy laughed. "I think I get it, you're not into expensive vitamins."

"All I am saying is that there are better things to spend your money on, like quality food, where you will get a much greater return on your money and on your health."

"Instead of spending $100 a month for fancy vitamins, spend $50 bucks and cover the whole year. Take the money you save each month and get some quality fish oil, and spend the rest of that money to eat healthy food. That money is better spent on natural or organic produce, free-range chicken, and grass-fed beef.

"Those are all topics we can discuss further down the road, though."

"Fine by me," said Timmy. "I have enough stuff to put into practice already."

"I think so too. I look forward to watching your progress over the coming weeks and months."

"Me too. I am excited to lose this weight. Every day just keeps getting better and better. I think I can be below 300 pounds by the time I leave for Thanksgiving."

"That is a great goal, Timmy!"

"Yeah, I am going to keep eating right and weighing myself every day."

"Hold on a second, you are going to do what?"

35

Don't Watch The Scale

"I am going to keep eating right," said Timmy as his eyes darted around the room.

"No, after that. What did you say?"

"Uh, that I was going to weigh myself every day," said Timmy sheepishly.

"Yes, that is what I thought I heard.

"I need to take a second here and tell you what I usually have to tell the women I work with. Women are usually the big culprits with this one, but I don't want you falling into that trap; the trap of watching the scale!"

Timmy laughed but avoided eye contact with Matthew.

"What is so wrong with scales, Matthew?"

"Nothing is wrong with scales. Scales are great; they just need to be used a lot less frequently than they are."

"What is the problem with getting on the scale every day?"

"The problem with stepping on the scale every day, especially for women, is that there are so many things that can cause 'weight' to fluctuate. As you learned earlier, it is easy to gain and lose water weight. If you are weighing yourself every day, a large part of your 'weight' fluctuations will be because of water, not fat loss.

"I try to get people to step on the scale only once or twice a month at first. That way, enough time passes so that no matter what is going on with water weight, the person can still see great results. Seeing results helps people to keep moving forward."

"I can see that. That makes sense."

"Here is another example. Let's say your sister starts eating right and even starts doing some working out. She steps on the scale before she starts and it says 140lbs. She works out for a few weeks and ate healthy over that time. Her clothes are fitting better and she likes the way things are going."

"I'm with you," said Timmy.

"Then she steps on the scale. It says 140 lbs. What? Both of us can hear the screams. 'How can that be? It isn't fair! I worked out hard, I ate right, and I haven't lost a pound!! ARGH. Forget it, I'm going to quit…'

"Can you see that, Timmy?"

Timmy nodded slowly. "Yes, I can see something like that happening."

"Here is the thing. The scale said she didn't lose any weight, but do you know what she DID do? She gained five pounds of muscle and lost five pounds of fat. So no, she didn't lose any weight, but she dramatically changed her body composition!"

"Really, how is that?"

"Did you know that a pound of body fat has 5x the volume as a pound of muscle?"

"Really? I had no idea. So that means that with all of my walking, I could have put some muscle on my legs, which means I have actually lost even more body fat?"

"That is a very possible, Timmy. Your muscles would have to grow with the amount of walking you have done lately. You went from a very sedentary lifestyle to one of movement. Not just hat, but your legs get a workout having to move 300 pounds all day long.

"Let's get back to the example with your sister for a second. No, the scale didn't move at all, but remember how she said her clothes were fitting better, and that she liked the way she was feeling?"

"Yes."

"Well, if those tangible things were making her feel so good, why would she let a number on a scale take that away and make her feel bad?"

"I don't know. You are right again, Matthew. I can see how similar things would apply to me."

"I won't even get into the fact that women's weight fluctuates ALL the time. That is largely due to the menstrual cycle and the hormones that wreak havoc on many women with regard to water retention.

"That said, my advice is to only check your weight once a week, or every ten days to two weeks if you can go that long. When you do check your weight, do it at the same time, preferably in the morning upon waking up, after you have used the rest room."

"Ok, I will weigh myself once a week at the most, and when I do check it, I will do it at the same time."

"Good. It doesn't do any good to check your weight one day first thing in the morning and then do it another time late in the day after you ate a salty meal for lunch that is causing you to retain water like a sham-wow. Got it?"

Timmy nodded in agreement.

"If for whatever reason you just can't break your grip on the scale, at least weigh yourself at the same time each day, and TRY to do it only a few times per week. It is much tougher to see progress when you are checking every day or a few times per week. You start doing things like not drinking water on certain days because you are thinking about the number on the scale, and that is not what we want."

"That makes perfect sense."

"If you do the things we have talked about, I guarantee that you will lose the weight. You don't need the scale to convince you of that. Your brother's comment when he first saw you should mean more to you than any number on a scale.

"He saw a difference. That is what we are after. Just wait until Thanksgiving when you are below 300 pounds. Your parents and sister are definitely going to recognize the fact that you will have lost over twenty-five pounds of body fat."

Timmy smiled. "I can't wait. Next stop 250!"

"I love your attitude. You really are going to be an inspiration to so many people."

"You think so?"

"I know so."

"Well, Timmy, it has been another great session. I have to run to a meeting, and I know you have class.

Have a great rest of the week, and call or email me if you have any questions along the way."

"Will do. Thanks, Matthew!

36

Letter to Mom #5 – "Times are a Changing"

Three more weeks have gone by, and Timmy has been on a role. He has been consistently eating 5 to 6 meals per day. Not only are his energy levels constant, but Matthew was right again; the pounds are really coming off.

Timmy knew Matthew was probably right, but there was still a part of him that didn't want to believe what he was hearing. For somebody that has always had a huge appetite, it was a stretch to believe that eating certain foods could naturally curb his appetite.

The thing is, it does work. Timmy never would have believed that drinking a glass of water with four to six almonds before a meal could make such a big difference. Eating fats, carbs, and protein in every meal was huge. Timmy was now a believer.

If he weren't a believer, the scale would have totally convinced him. In the past three weeks, Timmy had lost another ten pounds. He was very close to his goal of going home for Thanksgiving below 300 pounds, and he still had three weeks to go!

He was actually thinking he could be 295 or even 290 at the pace he had been going. The funny thing is that even though it was getting colder outside, Timmy kept walking. He was like the Forrest Gump of walkers. Not only did it allow him to clear his head and visualize the things he wanted to accomplish in life, but he was literally walking the pounds off.

Timmy had just finished another brisk walk around campus in the cold November air. He walked up the stairs to his apartment where he made a nice hot cup of green tea.

The warm tea felt so good going down his throat and into his stomach. It warmed his belly and put a smile on his face.

He grabbed his cup of tea, pulled out his laptop, and sat down in front of his computer.

Thursday, November 4

Dear Mom,

I know you are doing great, so I don't even have to ask. Things have been incredible since my last letter to you. I had a rough time at that football game, but I have turned that into a positive thing for me.

I emailed Matthew and told him I was ready to take things to the next level. He sat down with me and we spent a lot of time together. I learned so much about being healthy, and how the body works. It was totally eye opening.

I have to admit; I was very skeptical at first. I knew what he was telling me must be true, but part of me still had doubts; it's hard to change a decade of bad habits. On my way home that day, I saw a quote posted outside a teacher's office that said something to the effect of: "Doing the same thing over and over and expecting a different result is never going to work."

For the past three weeks, I have been doing exactly what Matthew taught me to do. I feel so much better, and everything he said, no matter how counterintuitive, turned out to be true. If my energy levels were lying to me, the scale sure wasn't. I lost another ten pounds in the past three weeks!

The thing that really amazes me is that it is so easy! It doesn't rely on self-control or depriving yourself. Trust me Mom, you know how big my appetite is. Matthew taught me a way to use food to control my appetite. The food tells my body to stop eating and to burn body fat.

I know it sounds crazy, but it works! You would truly be amazed if you saw the size of the meals that I am eating now. They are small compared to what you are used to seeing me eat, but the amazing thing is that they fill me up now!

I don't have time to go into all of it right now, but Matthew made a Keep It Simple sheet for me. I put a copy of it behind this letter. I can't wait to go over it with you when I come home for Thanksgiving. I can go into more depth and answer any questions you might have.

I can't wait to see you guys; it will only be three more weeks!

Well, I have to get some homework done and run to the grocery store. Seriously, read the KISS sheet (Keep It Super Simple) that I put with this letter.

Tell everybody that I am doing great and that I send lots of love!

Love you, Mom....

Little Timmy

37

When Life Deals Lemons, Start Making Lemonade

Thanksgiving was just around the corner. You know how it is in the days leading up to a big holiday weekend. Everybody is happy and ready to go spend time with friends and family. There is an energy present that normally isn't there.

Timmy had finished his last class and was looking forward to his walk back to the apartment. The sun was out, but the temperature had dropped pretty dramatically over the past few days. It was definitely cold out, and you could tell because very few people were braving the outdoors.

But Timmy was not one of those people. He was happy to get outside and walk. He knew he had hot green tea to warm his cold throat when he got home. Not only that, but he was on a mission to leave as much body fat as possible on campus before heading home for Thanksgiving.

He had already blown away his goal and was down to 292 pounds. This thought brought a smile to his face. Timmy took a second to make sure his cooler was secure in his backpack. Then he zipped his jacket and headed for the double doors that separated the cozy warm academic building from the harsh cold on the outside.

Timmy hit the escape handle with both hands and a resounding "thwack!" In an instant, he felt a 60-degree temperature change. His ears turned to ice before he was even down the steps in front of the building. He didn't care; he was happy and actually looking forward to taking the long way back.

The sidewalks were empty on this cold afternoon as most students opted to drive their cars around campus with the heat cranked up, but not Timmy.

He was walking down the sidewalk at a pace faster than most of the cars. The stop signs and speed bumps kept the cars inching along at a snail's pace while Timmy was working up a sweat as he walked briskly towards his apartment.

He was just thinking to himself how nice it was out. Yes, it was cold, but it wasn't like he lacked insulation, as he chuckled to himself. He was plenty warm, and his jacket was doing its job, even if it didn't fit as snug as it used to.

He was definitely flying by the cars now. As he approached a unique 3-way intersection where traffic always backed up, it happened.

There was a black Chevy Tahoe with tinted windows. The rear window slid down about half way and somebody yelled out, "Hey!"

Timmy turned to look over his right shoulder.

"You can walk all you want fat-boy, but you will always be fat! Do everybody a favor and try not to eat ALL the food over Thanksgiving break!! Ha-ha! Fat ass!"

Timmy stopped in his tracks. His mind was moving 100 miles per hour trying to assess the damage from the verbal daggers that impaled him. They were right. No they weren't, he told himself. Should he go confront them, or should he just keep walking? Part of him wanted to drop to the ground and just cry, another part wanted to fight, and another wanted to ignore them; but his body didn't move.

He thought about the weight he had lost, and that maybe the guy was right. He still had a good 100 pounds to lose. Maybe he would overeat at Thanksgiving. After all, he loved his mom's cooking.

He fought a mental battle for what seemed like forever, but it really lasted only about three seconds.

Timmy hung his head low, turned around, and kept walking. His pace was slower, and a blind man could've read the dejection in his body language.

He only made it about ten steps before he heard another voice.

"Hey, Timmy!"

He was hesitant to turn around after what just happened, but part of him thought he recognized the voice.

Then he heard the voice again.

"Hey Timmy, it's John…"

He thought to himself, there must be a God, because there were only one or two voices Timmy wanted to hear at that moment, and John's would have been one of those voices.

"…I'm with Matthew. We just heard what happened. Hop in, and come grab a coffee with us."

Timmy stopped in his tracks and lifted his gaze from the pavement in front of him just enough to see John behind the wheel with Matthew sitting in the passenger seat.

With his head still hanging low, Timmy walked across the street, threw his backpack across the seat and slid into the back of John's car.

Timmy kept his head low and tried to avoid eye contact with either John or Matthew. His eyes were shiny like glass as he was holding back a wall of tears. The last thing he wanted was for John and Matthew to see him like this, but at the same time if anybody would be able to help him, it would be them.

John spoke first. "Timmy, as you know, I used to be very overweight myself. I used to get the looks, stares, and comments all the time. I know from being in your shoes that there is nothing that Matthew or myself can say to take the pain away, or truly make you feel better.

"I know it isn't easy, and it might take some time, but the best way to deal with people and situations like that is to have a strong mind and self-confidence. I know that is especially hard because you say to yourself, 'I'm still fat; I'm not where I want to be yet. I will have confidence when I lose X more pounds.'

"But I am telling you, self-confidence isn't based on a weight. It is based on how you see yourself. It is based on how you visualize yourself. I know you have been doing your visualizations and working on your mindset, as both Matthew and I have noticed a huge change in you."

"We really have," chimed in Matthew.

"You used to be this extremely timid guy that wondered, 'Why would anybody want to talk to me?' I saw it, Matthew saw it, and my assistant, Sandy, saw it. But over the past three months, you have transformed yourself.

"It isn't just a physical transformation of losing weight, but your mind has shifted. I have overheard your interactions with Matthew, I have seen you walking taller and with more confidence. Sandy even mentioned your interaction with her when you needed copies made recently.

"You know you have come a long way, and you know you are going to end up achieving your goals. I know it hurts, but you can't let the words of some insecure stranger derail all of your progress and hard work."

Timmy sat in the back seat but slowly picked his head up to look into the rear view mirror to see John's face.

His eyes met John's in the mirror. Timmy gave a slow nod.

"I was just minding my own business, enjoying a brisk walk back to my apartment. I was happy, just thinking about how nice it was going to be when I see my family in two days."

"I know you were," said John. "What that person did wasn't right, but it is up to you if those words have an impact or not."

Timmy nodded in agreement. "Honestly, the pain is going away. I think I was just in shock more than anything else. I know that people will still look at me right now as being overweight, but they have no idea how far I have come."

"I know, Timmy, I have been there. Sadly, there will always be insecure people that will say mean things, no matter what you look like physically.

"That is why you can't say you will get self-confidence at a certain weight. Sure, I know it helps, but confidence comes from the inside. You might be a normal weight and nobody is calling you 'fat,' but that isn't going to mean you have any amount of self-confidence; that comes from within," said John.

Matthew nodded his head. "Timmy, remember what your brother said about me at the football game? I know it is different, but I only point it out so that you can see that no matter what, there will always be people out there that will feel the need to put others down to make themselves feel better."

Timmy looked at Matthew. "I understand, but isn't it easier to deal with that because you are in good shape?"

"It can be easier, but no matter what, you have to have the self confidence from within to not let it bother you. As human beings, we generally want other people to like or at least respect us just as another human being. Why would anybody want to 'put down' a complete stranger they don't even know?"

"Because of their own insecurity?" said Timmy timidly.

"Exactly," said Matthew.

"Believe it or not, Timmy, some of the most insecure people in the world are people you would never expect: celebrities, movie stars, athletes, and models. They might look like they have it all together, but many are looking outwardly for acceptance because they don't have self-confidence on the inside."

With that, something clicked in his head. In a split second, Timmy actually understood what Matthew was talking about. "So you are saying they are constantly looking outwardly to things like fame and the media for validation since they don't have it on the inside?"

"That is it," said Matthew.

"I know this is going to be a challenge for you, Timmy. Even when I reached my normal weight, I still saw myself as overweight. It was a difficult battle I had to fight. The first step in that battle is awareness," said John.

"Once you are aware that you are doing it, you can stop yourself. It is not being aware that makes it easier to spiral downward and go back to your old ways. We have seen so many people give up because of a setback, or because they internalized something that was said to them.

"If you believe what others say, it becomes true for you. How can you succeed when a hammer is always falling on your head? When people say mean things, that is their issue, not yours; so don't buy it! With education and persistence, you will win the war.

"The second step is eliminating the limiting beliefs and replacing them with positive ones you know are true."

Timmy managed to look up at John.

"The third step is anchoring that new belief about yourself into your current reality. Some suggest hanging a picture of your 'old,' 325 pound self on the fridge to remind you of where you came from. We believe you should be motivated by the positive outlook of the future, as opposed to using fear generated by the past.

"One way to solidify your new belief is to find a picture that represents the body you want to have. Paste a picture of your head onto that body, put it on the fridge, and carry it around with you everywhere you go. Let this picture become ingrained into your mind. Visualize it. It will serve as a constant reminder of your success and where you are headed in life."

Timmy was now sitting up straight. His eyes were no longer glossed over like a glass dam holding back a wall of tears.

John swung his car into the parking lot of the local coffee shop. He parked away from the door and other cars. He turned the car off and turned to Timmy.

"Are you ready to go in? We can take a few more minutes if you would like. I know the place gets crowded on days like today."

"Actually, I'm fine. Your words were very powerful and make so much sense. I'm not sure I would have been able to fight that mentally by myself. Not only did your talk help, but I love your ideas for handling negative encounters going forward.

"I actually think I am stronger because of it. That is the first time in a while somebody has been vocal to me. I am over the people staring, or looking out of the corner of their eye, but that situation really took me by surprise.

"If anything, it just motivates me even more.

"That said; I have a question."

"What is it?" replied John.

"Where can I get a picture of Matthew's body?" asked Timmy with a big grin on his face.

They all three laughed.

"So, which one of you is buying my green tea today?" said Timmy as he opened the car door.

Matthew managed to stop laughing long enough to say, "I got it. Don't worry about it, Timmy."

"It is really good to see you taking this so well," said John. "There was a time when a similar thing happened to me, and it took me days to get over it. I was so angry inside."

"Let's get inside and enjoy ourselves," said Matthew.

The coffee shop was pretty crowded, but the three of them were able to find a table as a group was leaving. John and Timmy sat down as Matthew went to order.

"John, I really can't thank you enough. If it wasn't for you, and introducing me to Matthew, I don't know what would have happened to me. I do know that there is no way in the world I would be almost 290 pounds. Can you believe that I have lost almost 30 pounds?"

John put his hand on Timmy's shoulder and looked him in the eye. "You did it Timmy; all we did was provide you with some guidance and information. You have no idea how happy it makes us to see people actually commit to taking the actions we suggest.

"We work with so many people, and you would be amazed at how many people just quit and never follow through. It is people like you that make this job so rewarding. Matthew and I talk about you a lot. You really are an inspiration, Timmy."

"Here you go, guys," said Matthew as he placed the beverages on the table.

"Green tea for Timmy, chai tea for me, and John, your favorite mocha macchiato."

The three of them sat there and talked for a few minutes, and the topic finally landed on Thanksgiving plans.

"Are you looking forward to seeing your family?" John asked Timmy.

"You bet I am! I can't wait to see my mom and my sister especially. I miss them the most."

"Any big plans while you are home?"

"Not really, it's just going to be nice to see Mom outside of the hospital and spend time with the family.

"The only thing I am sort of worried about is the Thanksgiving meal. As you know, my family likes to eat. Most Thanksgivings we usually have a 'who has to loosen their belt the most' contest.

"Fortunately, I don't feel like winning, much less competing this year," said Timmy, cracking a smile.

Matthew and John both laughed.

"Remember, Thanksgiving is just another meal," said Matthew. "You don't have to eat all that food at once, it isn't going anywhere. The beauty is that Thanksgiving usually provides delicious food for many meals in the form of leftovers.

"Just keep doing what you have been doing. Keep eating your snacks or mini-meals, as it will help you to not be starving when the moment arrives.

"I love Thanksgiving because I can make so many healthy meals out of the leftovers. So for me, it is about way more than one tasty meal, it is about multiple meals spread out over a few days. So keep that mindset and you won't feel the pressure to eat it all on Thanksgiving Day."

"That makes perfect sense. I like that idea!" exclaimed Timmy. A huge smile crossed his face, "I can use the leftover turkey as the protein for several meals."

"That's what I'm talking about," said Matthew.

All of a sudden, Timmy's face got pale white. He stopped talking and his eyes were frozen in a gaze over Matthew's right shoulder as if he had seen a ghost.

"What is it, Timmy?" asked John.

Matthew turned to look over his shoulder. It took him a second to figure out what had made Timmy freeze like a deer in headlights.

When he saw what it was, he turned around completely.

"Hey, Natalie!"

"Oh hey, Matthew!"

"Get your coffee, then come over here for a second."

"Sure thing," said Natalie.

Timmy's eyes were as wide as the dinner plates he used to eat on.

"What are you doing?" asked Timmy forcefully.

"What? I am just inviting a friend over to say 'hi.' Do you have a problem with that?"

Timmy couldn't even muster a response. All the blood had rushed out of his face and hands, so he grabbed his hot tea and wrapped both hands around it for warmth.

"Hi, Matthew, how are you doing? Nice day, but definitely getting that winter chill in the air," said Natalie.

"Yes, definitely getting cold out, but thankfully the snow is holding off for now. I am doing great. I believe you have met John before."

"Yes, I have." Natalie reached out to shake his hand. "Nice to see you again."

"But I don't think you have met Timmy."

Natalie extends her hand. "Hi, Timmy, nice to meet you."

Timmy continued to grasp that hot cup of tea with all of his might. It was the only thing keeping his hands from trembling.

"You can do this. Be strong. You are the kind of person people want to know. You are popular. You have a lot to offer." All of the affirmations and things Timmy had visualized were flowing through his head. "I can do this," he thought.

In what seemed like an eternity, but in reality was only a split second, Timmy managed to pry his right hand off the cup of tea. Amazingly, his hand was no longer shaking and twitching and he extended it to meet Natalie's.

"Very nice to meet you," said Timmy, but not quite bringing his eyes up to meet hers'.

"Do you have a second? Want to sit down and join us?" inquired Matthew.

"Sure, I would love to!"

Natalie happily sat down at the table. John and Matthew made eye contact and a slight smile crossed both of their faces, as they knew this was a big step for Timmy.

Timmy on the other had was trying to act "normal" in the face of what seemed like a tidal wave of terror coming right towards him.

"So John and I have been working with Timmy here for the past few months. His mom had a heart attack and he came to us for help as he saw himself heading down that same path."

"He has already lost about thirty pounds, and he has really been an inspiration to us," said Matthew.

"That is awesome," exclaimed Natalie, as she reached out and put her hand on Timmy's arm.

It was like electricity shooting through his body. He had never felt anything like that before. He was literally in shock, but somehow managed to keep his composure.

"My dad was extremely overweight and battled heart disease for years," said Natalie.

The tidal wave of fear was slowly dissipating. "Really? Somebody in your family battled weight issues?"

"Yes. My mom is healthy, but Dad buried himself in work. He ate out all the time for business lunches and dinners and never worked out. Over the years, that lifestyle took a toll on him until he found himself in the hospital. I can totally relate to your experience."

Timmy raised his head a bit more and finally managed to make eye contact with Natalie. In that moment, he realized he had nothing to fear from those beautiful blue eyes, or in anybody's eyes for that matter. In fact, her eyes had a calming effect on him.

"We have been working with Timmy on changing his lifestyle and giving him healthy habits he can use for the rest of his life," said Matthew.

"That is just great," said Natalie. "You know, I have seen you walking around campus. You are literally always walking, no matter what temperature it is outside."

"Yeah, that's me," said Timmy as a crease formed in his cheek and a slightly nervous grin crossed his face. "Matthew said I needed to walk if I wanted to lose the weight, so I just started walking everywhere. The thing is, I actually enjoy it now."

"That is great," said Natalie. "Mind if I walk with you sometime if we're heading the same way?"

Timmy didn't know what to say. His mouth was dry as the Sahara, and his tongue was frozen like the Arctic. He slowly nodded his head as a smile began to overtake his cheeks.

"Sh…sh…sure, that would be great," stammered Timmy.

"Perfect. Well, you guys have a great holiday. I have to run. And Timmy, I'm serious about the walk."

Natalie smiled at the three of them, touched Timmy on the shoulder, and turned to walk away. As she turned, she gave Matthew a wink, which was returned with the slightest nod of acknowledgement.

Timmy just sat there with the biggest smile on his face. Not only did he meet somebody new, but it was a girl, and not just any girl; it was Natalie Williams.

"In the past hour, I think I experienced one of the lowest lows, and one of the highest-highs of my life," exclaimed Timmy. "Matthew, at first I wanted to kill you for calling her over. I was terrified, but you know, she is just a regular person."

"That is the point, Timmy. There really is nothing to be scared of. All of the fear is of your own creation in your mind. As your self-confidence increases, you will realize you have nothing to be afraid of."

"Huh. That kind of reminds me of something my grandmother used to say about fear—that it's just 'false evidence appearing real.' You are right about all that. Not only was Natalie nice and down to earth, but she actually noticed me walking around campus! "

John and Matthew smiled and nodded at Timmy.

"I feel great! I just want to thank you guys for everything that you have done for me. I appreciate it more than you could possibly know."

Timmy finished his cup of tea and pushed it towards the center of the table.

"I know you both have other things to do, and I want to hit the grocery to pick up a few things before it gets too dark out. But I just want to say thanks again. You both really are amazing."

"You're welcome, Timmy. Are you sure you don't want a ride?" John asked.

"That's ok, John. I really appreciate it, but I would rather walk. "That reminds me; I meant to ask this earlier. Matthew, what else can I do as far as working out? Any workouts or anything I can do?"

"Of course there are things you can do. We will start covering more of the physical aspect of working out once we come back next semester. That will give you some more time to make these habits permanent, as well as lose more weight, which will make you much less likely to get injured."

"That makes sense, but anything in the meantime?"

"Well, there are three things you can do," said Matthew. "Modified push-ups, modified squats, and arm circles.

"For the modified push-ups, start by placing your feet two to three feet away from a wall. Lean towards the wall with your hands in front of you at about shoulder height or a little bit lower. Place your palms on the wall shoulder width apart, and bend your elbows and move your chest towards the wall, then push away.

"Start by doing ten to twelve repetitions and work your way up to three sets of twenty. Once that is easy, you are going to transition from using the wall to a counter top.

"Let me guess, I am going to progress to where eventually I can do a push-up?"

"Exactly."

"It will probably take you a while to get to that point, so stick to the wall and counter push-ups for the next month or so at least. When you get good at the counter push-ups, you can always do more sets and reps.

"I want you to talk with me before you try knee push-ups or regular push-ups. You need to lose some weight before you can put your weight on your knees. Again, we don't want to get you injured."

"Makes sense, Matthew. I will stick to just doing wall and counter push-ups for a while. What about squats?"

"For squats, I want you to find a stable chair that has arms. I want you sit down with your back straight, not touching the back of the chair. Use the arms of the chair to assist you as you stand up. You should be focusing on using your legs like this." Matthew did a quick demonstration as he got up out of his chair.

"I got it. How many should I do?"

"Work on doing ten to fifteen reps for three sets. Feel free to do this multiple times per day if you wish. The important thing is to do it injury free. So start slow, and just work your way up.

"Lastly, do arm circles. Put your arms out to the side and make small circles forward. Work up to 30 seconds, then rest. Then do small circles backwards.

"The small circles will be the size of a large orange, and the bigger circles will be the size of a medium pizza. Does that make sense?"

"That makes sense. So do small forward for 30 seconds, rest, small back for 30 seconds, rest, and then do the same thing with bigger circles."

"You got it! Feel free to call or email me if you have any questions. Keep walking, and add those three exercises during the day. As you lose more weight, there will be more exercises that we can do where there is a very low risk of injury.

"Another thing you can do is go walk stairs or hills. It is a great workout, just be careful coming down too fast. Try to keep a steady and balanced pace both up and down the hill; you never want to be out of control. When in doubt, slow down."

"Sounds like a plan. Well, thanks for those quick tips, Matthew. I am going to head to the grocery and then home. Have a great Thanksgiving and I will see both of you next week!"

Timmy stood up from the table and remembered that his bag was in John's car. "John, can I get my bag out of your car?"

"Sure. Let me walk out with you so you can get it."

"Thanks, John."

John and Timmy walked outside to the car so he could get his belongings. Matthew sat at the table and took a sip of his chai tea with a big smile on his face. Watching Timmy progress really made him happy.

He just knew Timmy would be successful in life. In all the years Matthew had been helping people, he had seen one characteristic that all successful students had, and that was desire.

The desire to succeed had to be greater than the pain of doing nothing. It was obvious Timmy had the desire. You could see it in his eyes, hear it in his voice, and it was starting to show in the way he carried himself.

Matthew was looking forward to watching the complete transformation of Timmy.

38

Home for Thanksgiving

The last time Timmy made this drive was to see his mom in the hospital. Fortunately, he was making this trip under much happier circumstances, the long Thanksgiving weekend.

Timmy grabbed his cooler and stocked it with an assortment of snacks for the trip. Even though there would be plenty of food at home, he knew that staying on track would be much easier if he had his cooler with him.

He had worked hard to make this new routine a habit, and he wasn't about to blow it over a long holiday weekend, especially one that typically involved stuffing oneself to the point of discomfort.

Timmy tossed his bag in the trunk and put his cooler in the passenger seat. He stood there for a second looking at his filthy car that hadn't been washed in months. He just looked at it and smiled, as the filth symbolized how little he had driven lately.

Driving had been replaced by walking, and don't worry, unlike his car, he took a shower at least once a day.

Before sliding into the car, he stared at the well-worn driver's seat that looked quite different from the passenger seat. It was a constant reminder of the weight he had been carrying around.

Timmy promised himself that he wouldn't even think of getting a new car until he was below 200 pounds. He knew that could easily be at least a year, but it would serve as good motivation for him.

He sat down in his Chevy Cavalier, turned the key, and the car sputtered to life. The cold weather and lack of being driven lately meant the car needed a few seconds get going, and a minute or so until it reached a smooth idle.

Timmy put the car in drive and began his trip home.

He turned the radio off and was just alone with his thoughts. A lot had happened in the past few months, and Timmy was just going over it all in his head.

Then it hit him. He remembered the part of his last trip when he made his promise to God. Timmy said he would do anything if God would just make his mom healthy. Maybe Matthew was right, maybe he was going to help a lot of people. He sure had learned a lot, and maybe he could start by sharing some much needed information with his loved ones.

Matthew said Timmy was going to be an ambassador, but he just assumed that meant for overweight people, but maybe it could be God?

Timmy's mind was racing. "Maybe God put John and Matthew in my life so that I would be the one that finally motivated Mom to get healthy. Maybe I am supposed to help others that are overweight."

It didn't matter why it happened. The thing is, it did happen, and Timmy wasn't going to waste this opportunity. He made up his mind right then and there that he was going to not only lose his weight, but be that outgoing person that others would look up to.

He saw the joy in John and Matthew's faces when they looked at his progress. His success made them happy, and he badly wanted to help others the way they had helped him.

A road sign off to the side caught his eye. "I can't believe it," he thought to himself. This trip is flying by, and I am almost home.

Timmy stopped at the local gas station by his house as he was almost on empty. He smiled and shook his head as he looked through the windows and saw the shelves lined with junk food.

The old Timmy would have taken five bucks inside to get some Zingers, Cheetos, and soda, but the new Timmy was no longer craving junk food. Instead, he finished filling his car and sat back down in the driver's seat to eat a few apple slices with peanut butter on them.

He polished it off with a protein drink he had made before he left. The last thing Timmy wanted was to show up at home with an appetite.

Finally, he swung his car around 180 degrees to park on the street in front of his house. He climbed out of the car and headed for the front door.

As he approached the front door, he could see and smell the smoke that was billowing out of the fireplace. It made him happy to be home.

Just as Timmy was reaching to put his key in the door, it opened. There was Mom standing there wearing her cooking apron and a smile.

The sight of his mom sent a smile beaming across his face.

"Oh my God, Timmy! You look great! Come here, give me a hug!"

Timmy couldn't get a word in as Susan wrapped her arms around Timmy and just kept squeezing him relentlessly like a boa constrictor with its prey. She grabbed his arms with both hands and pushed her body back so she could get a good look at her boy.

"I can't believe how much weight you have lost, young man! You look amazing! I have really enjoyed all of your letters, but I have to tell you, I was somewhat skeptical that it would work, or that you would stick with it."

Timmy smiled confidently.

"Your face, oh my. How much weight have you lost?"

"I have already lost over thirty pounds, with another 100 to go until I reach my goal weight."

"Wow, I am so proud of you. I have lost about eight pounds myself, but you are an inspiration to me. If you can do it, so can I!"

Timmy slowly backed his mom up out of the doorway so that he could close the door. After all, it was freezing outside.

"I want to sit down with you and hear about everything you have learned. This family needs to make some changes, and I think whatever you have been doing looks like the place to start."

"Everybody, guess who is home!" shouted Susan over her shoulder.

The family congregated by the front door to welcome Timmy home. Every one of them was in awe of not just the weight that

Timmy had lost, but also a newfound energy and purpose about him that they sensed.

Timmy didn't get much time to relax, as Susan and the rest of the family wanted to hear about everything he had learned the past few months.

He managed to hold them off for a few minutes so that he could get his things out of the car and make some hot green tea.

Timmy sat down with the entire family and told them the story that was the past few months. No detail was spared as he told them the ups and downs he had encountered. Timmy beamed with excitement as he recounted the challenges and the successes.

When he was finished, Susan said, "I want to know more!"

"Well," said Timmy with a chuckle. "I told you everything I know at the moment. John and Matthew have a lot more to teach me, and I have a lot more to learn. Look at the bright side, you will have something to look forward to each day when you go and check the mail."

"You know I like surprises," said Susan, beaming with pride.

"Remember, I still have 100 pounds to lose, and they have so many things they want to teach me as the time comes. From fitness, to finances, to relationships, this is only the beginning. The cool thing is that everything they teach me will apply to the rest of my life!"

"Well I'll be," said Susan. "I look forward to more."

"That said, after listening to Timmy for the past few hours, and seeing how much weight he has lost, I think we will do Thanksgiving a bit differently tomorrow."

"What do you mean?" asked Jason.

"Well, a couple of things. Timmy has worked so hard to lose weight; I want to keep that going. So I won't be pushing people to 'eat up' tomorrow. In fact, after hearing about how he eats five or six times per day, I think we should have our main meal at lunchtime, and spread the leftovers out over the rest of the day."

"That actually sounds like a great idea," said Jessica. "I am all for it. I think we can all stand to adopt healthier habits as a family."

Everybody nodded in agreement, except for Don.

"You guys do what you want. This is my favorite holiday, and I am not going to let some diet that somebody else is trying ruin it for me."

"Timmy, if you want to nibble like a little girl and eat your little fruit and nut snacks out of plastic baggies, go ahead. But I'm a real man, and I eat real man food, in real man sized portions. Right, Jason? You're with me on this. You said yourself you don't think Timmy will be able to lose weight."

Jason looked away, avoiding any eye contact with Timmy.

Susan gasped.

Jessica dropped her fork.

Timmy was stunned.

He really thought everyone in his own family would be more supportive. And Jason, why would he say such hurtful things behind his back? After all, he left such a nice note, and had even met Matthew.

But Timmy remembered what Matthew had said about how people react when they are unsure of themselves and understood that it must be difficult for Jason to be stuck in the middle.

Timmy stood up, a lump forming in his throat and placed his hand on Don's shoulder.

"Dad, I love you. You have raised me well and I respect you for that. I have no right to come in here and ask you to change how you have been doing things in your life in your own house. You can eat the way that you want and it doesn't matter to me. I still love you no matter what you eat."

Timmy paused for a second.

"But I also know that Grandpa died not too long ago at age sixty-five from heart disease. I just don't want to lose you Dad…like you lost your dad. Your life impacts more people than you know. It just hurts because you won't do something as simple and proven as eating better."

Don mumbled something under his breath, got off his Lazyboy chair, looked at Susan, and left the room. Timmy and the family looked at each other, not knowing what to do. Jason started to go after Don but Susan put her hand up.

"Let him be. He needs to be alone."

"Is he ok?" asked Timmy.

"No," countered Susan. "But he will be, in time."

Don sat in his car and took out the only picture he had of him with his dad. A tear rolled off his check and landed on the steering wheel. He missed his dad so much; the times they laughed, the times they went fishing together, but most of all watching him play with Jason, Timmy, and Jessica.

But his dad was gone now. Don wanted nothing more than to be there when his grandchildren graduated, get married, and had kids of their own. In his heart of hearts, he knew that Timmy was right.

Don went back inside the house and found Susan sitting alone in the family room with her head buried in her arms, recipe books and photo albums strewn all around. Don sat next to her and gently wrapped his hands around hers. Together they sat in silence.

Susan looked up at Don and into the eyes of a loving man whom she knew desperately wanted to live. Neither of them knew what the future had in store for them, but they both knew their fate if they continued down the same path.

Breaking the silence, Don stood to add more logs to the hot simmering coals. The fire sparked to life, causing Don to take a step back. As the blaze grew stronger, the fresh firewood crackled in earnest, making the Johnston house just a little bit brighter than before.

39

FitLife212 – Lifestyle Coaching: It's All About You

I have some good news for you, but before we get going, I need you to do something for me.

Take a break and stop thinking about the kids, family, work, deadlines, or whatever else is on your mind. I want you to be selfish for a few minutes, because we are going to take some time and focus on your favorite person…you!

You are reading this for a reason, so let's get right to the point.

FitLife212 Lifestyle Coaching & Consulting is designed to give you the power, but more importantly, a framework to change your lifestyle so that you get what you want out of life. The beauty of this system is that it revolves around and is focused on **your** specific wants, goals, and desires. Your end result or goal can be completely different from your friend's or even society's, but that doesn't matter. What matters is that you get what you want, and that is what separates this system from the rest…it is all about you!

Things you will learn

- Have you ever wished somebody would accompany you to the grocery store and teach you how to read labels and shop for food?

- Does all the marketing hype make understanding food labels hard?
- Do you ever feel overwhelmed by the amount of "diet," health, and fitness information on the internet, in the news, and elsewhere?
- Are you tired of diets, quick fixes, and "magic pills" that don't work?
- Would you like to lose weight, keep it off, and never have to diet again?

If you answered yes to any of these questions, then lifestyle coaching could be a perfect solution for you. Imagine living a lifestyle where you are happy with your body, enjoying the activities you like to do, and most importantly, eating the foods you like to eat.

Where the mind goes, the body will follow.

The first step will be to answer five short questions. You will keep these answers by your bed and look at them before you go to sleep and first thing when you wake up. In addition, from these five questions we will make three short sentences that you can review throughout the day. Put it on your computer or the refrigerator door. Doesn't matter where you put it, just so long as you can see it to help keep you on track.

Structure – A Framework for Action & Success

Are you one of those people that do better with structure in place? I know, I know, we all like our freedom, but let's be honest, I believe we all do better with a plan in place. Why is the plan so important, you ask?

Simple. Comes down to one word: action.

It takes 17 to 30 days to create a new habit or change an old one. When a structure and plan is in place, it makes it easier for you to take action and get results. Procrastination, fear, and doubt have a much harder time showing up when you are on a mission and don't have time for distractions.

It is the difference between reading a book on a friend's recommendation and reading the travel guidebook you bought for your vacation that starts in a month. The vacation becomes the structure that nudges you to take action by actually reading the book before you leave. Since there is no timeframe for reading your friend's book suggestion, it probably won't get done (just being honest).

How many times have you set out to do something but never started, much less, completed, the task? It's ok, you can admit it. Almost everybody on the planet has done this at one time or another.

Millions of people have set out to read a book, lose weight, or learn a skill only to never end up doing it because they didn't have a structure in place to keep them on track.

Don't get me wrong here; I am not talking about a crazy inflexible structure. I am talking about a framework of positive reinforcement that will help keep you on track so that you get the things in life that you want.

This coaching program is designed to provide you structure along the way so that you succeed! Everybody starts out motivated, but that self-produced motivation can fade quickly or die completely at the first bump in the road. This coaching was designed so this doesn't happen, and you don't have to rely on just your inner fortitude to be successful.

I want you to stay on track and will be there to provide support and motivation along the way. Hey, we all have bad days. No need to let a bad day take you completely off course. I believe that you will really enjoy and respond to the subtle, and not so subtle, ways the system keeps you on track and in a positive state of mind!

Surround Yourself with Supportive People

Having supportive people go through the coaching with you makes things even easier for you on your path to success. This part is optional, but if you are really serious about getting what you want out of life, then you will take this step.

The more people in your circle of influence that commit to living a healthier lifestyle means faster and greater results for all involved. Who doesn't like to have a support system they can look to for help, motivation, or just to talk to?

Imagine if your family members, close friends, co-workers, or even entire company decided to adopt the core principles you will learn. How much easier would it be to succeed if you were surrounded by positive influences that were not testing your willpower at every turn? Wouldn't it be nice if you weren't being pressured to eat unhealthy food when going out for a meal?

Sure, it would take a little effort to share this with your friends, family, or co-workers, but can you imagine how it would feel to not only have those people there to support you, but also take on a leadership role in helping others? It is more powerful than you might think, and you would be surprised at what it will do for your confidence and the results you will achieve!

Either way, I am sure you can agree that having others there to help is a very positive thing. It shouldn't come as any surprise that having the proper environment can make the path to success easier. Not only that, but it removes the pressure of having to do it all on your own.

The Next Steps

Step 1 – Complete the 3-page handout titled 'Step1 - What Is Important To You?' Don't worry, there are no right or wrong answers, and it doesn't even take much writing, unless you want it to. Make sure you fill this form out by hand.

Step 2 – This one is really easy. Look at the list of foods in the handout and circle the foods you actually LIKE to eat. Not the foods you are supposed to like, but the foods that you would choose for yourself if nobody were around.

Step 3 – Take those sheets, combined with the special information you will learn from me, and put them into action. Once you see what I have in store for you, I think you will be surprised how easy it will be.

Step 4 – Continue taking action for TWO weeks. I have found that this two-week mark is a crucial point for most people. Get here and the odds are overwhelmingly in your favor that you will make a permanent change to your lifestyle habits.

Congratulations! You just took action by reading this far. For some of you, this might not be a big deal, but for many of you, taking this small action is a big step forward. Now that you know a bit about what is in store, let's get started with the coaching as we work together to create and adopt new, healthier, lifestyle habits for you.

I am looking forward to accompanying you as you take action and create a lifestyle that will lead to a happier, healthier, and more fulfilling life.

Remember: "Little things over time make a BIG difference!"

Best of luck on your Lean Life journey,

Brooks Hollan
FitLife212.com

Step 1 - What Is Important to You

The first thing you need to understand is that success with The Lean Life program is all about **you**. It is about your wants and desires; not society's, not your family's, not your friends', just yours.

The first step in achieving your goals is to figure out what they are and write them down. To help you with this, we have provided some questions for you to answer about yourself and your reasons for wanting to change your life.

The Lean Life system is designed to be simple. We have stripped away all the distractions and are going to focus on making this as easy as possible to implement in your life.

By answering these few simple questions, it will help provide the clarity and motivation for you on your path to living a new, healthier, and fulfilling life.

Take as much time as you need to answer the following 5 questions.

1. What is your primary reason for wanting to lose weight, be healthy, & adopt a healthy lifestyle?

We will help you get started on this first one. Is it so you can play with your kids or grandkids? Is it because you want to be able to walk a flight of stairs without being out of breath? Is it because you want to live longer? Is it because you had the life-long dream of running a marathon? Remember, there are no right or wrong answers; it is all about what is important to you.

_____

_____

_____

_____

_____

2. Why is this reason so important to you?

_____
_____
_____
_____
_____

3. How will losing weight & changing your lifestyle impact your life?

_____
_____
_____
_____
_____

4. Make a list of people you feel will offer support on your road to a Lean Life. These are typically your family, friends, or co-workers. These are the people you will want to surround yourself with, as the more support you have, the less you have to rely on willpower, and the easier it will be for you to achieve your goals.

_____
_____
_____
_____
_____

5. Once you have made a successful transformation and started living a Lean Life, name 5 people you would like to see make positive changes in their own lives. This is where you can become a role model and help others that were in your same situation.

1. _____

2. _____

3. _____

4. _____

5. _____

Keep the answers to these questions close to your bed. Review them on a daily basis. Read them before you go to bed at night and first thing in the morning when you wake up.

The more you review the reasons why this is important to you, the easier it will be for you to accomplish your goals. As you review the answers to these questions on a daily basis, your mindset will change. Your mind will begin to operate in a positive state instead of a state of negativity or doubt.

To help you even further, on the next page, there is a shorter version you can fill out and put on your desk, on the refrigerator, or any other place you see often that will help keep you focused. Plus, the repetition helps ingrain it in your mind.

I Am Going To Live a Lean Life Because…

The primary reason I want to lose weight is

_____

_____

_____

This reason is important to me because

_____

_____

_____

This reason will impact my life by

_____

_____

_____

I AM CHANGE

I AM A SUCCESS

I ACCOMPLISH MY GOALS

I AM A FAT-BURNING MACHINE

I AM LIVING A LEAN LIFE

I AM A ROLE MODEL

I AM A LEADER

Step 2 - Food: What I Like To Eat

The purpose of this sheet is to figure out what you like to eat. There is no pressure, and nobody is looking over your shoulder, so only circle the foods that you actually LIKE to eat. We are going to work together and use this information to make it super easy for you to create your own meals and mini-meals.

Listed below are some common foods that have been split into four groups. Circle the foods in each group that you like. If you don't see something on the list, write it in below the list where it says "Other." Use these foods with the "KISS Handout" and the info you will learn during your coaching.

Group 1

Beef – Lean Cuts
   Top Sirloin
   Strip Steak
   Top Round Steak
   Round Roast
   T-Bone Steak
   Flank Steak
   Tri-tip
Bison
Chicken Breast
Cottage Cheese (low Fat)
Egg – Whole
Egg Whites
Tofu

Fish –
Eat Unlimited
   Anchovies
   Catfish
   Clam
   Crab
   Crawfish
   Flounder
   Haddock
   Herring
   Mackerel

Mullet
Oyster
Perch
Pollock
Salmon
Sardine
Scallop
Shrimp
Sole
Squid
Tilapia
Trout
Tuna (Canned light)
Whitefish

Few times per week
   Bass
   Carp
   Cod
   Halibut
   Lobster
   Mahi Mahi
   Monkfish
   Perch
   Snapper

Few times per month
   Bluefish
   Bluefin
   Grouper
   Pike
   Sea Bass
   Shark
   Swordfish
   Tuna - Albacore
   Tuna - Yellowfin

Pork – lean cuts
   Pork Loin
   Loin Chops
   Tenderloin

Turkey Breast

Greek Yogurt – 2%
Greek Yogurt - Fat Free
Milk – 2%
Milk – Skim
Whey Protein Powder
Yogurt – 2%
Yogurt – Fat Free

Group 2
Circle your favorite foods:

Apple	Fig	Orange
Apricot	Gooseberry	Peach
Banana	Grape	Pear
Bilberry	Grapefruit	Pineapple
Black Currant	Guava	Plum
Blackberry	Honeydew	Pomegranate
Blueberry	Huckleberry	Prune
Cantaloupe	Kiwi	Raisin
Cherry	Kumquat	Raspberry
Clementine	Lemon	Redcurrant
Currant	Lime	Rhubarb
Date	Lychee	Strawberry
Durian	Mango	Tangerine
Eggplant	Nectarine	Watermelon

Artichoke	Chives	Olives
Asparagus	Collards	Peppers
Acorn Squash	Cucumber	Parsnip
Beets	Dandelion	Pickles
Bell Pepper	Dill Pickle	Radish
Black-eyed Peas	Edamame	Rutabaga
Broccoli	Eggplant	Romaine Lettuce
Brussels Sprouts	Garlic	Spinach
Butternut Squash	Ginger	Squash
Cauliflower	Green beans	Sprouts
Cabbage	Habanero Pepper	Spring Greens
Carrots	Jalapeno Pepper	Snow Peas
Celery	Kale	Tomato
Cilantro	Lettuce	Turnips
Cherry tomato	Mushrooms	Wasabe
Chili Pepper	Onions	Water chestnut
Chickpea	Okra	Yams
Chilies		Zucchini

Others:

Group 3
Circle your favorites:

Amaranth	Millet	Rice - White
Barley	Noodles (any kind)	Rye
Beans	Oats	Soybeans
Bread (whole grain)	Pasta (any kind)	Spelt
Couscous	Potato (any kind)	Sweet Potato
Whole-wheat pasta	Quinoa	Wheat berries
Flaxseed	Rice - Brown	Wild rice

Note: Generally, the less refined or processed a food is, the better.

Others:

Group 4

Almonds	Grape Seed Oil	Peanut Oil
Avocado	Guacamole	Pecans
Brazil nuts	Hazelnuts	Pine nuts
Canola Oil	Macadamia nuts	Pistachios
Cashews	Olive Oil	Pumpkin Seeds
Chestnuts	Olives	Sesame Seeds
Coconut Oil	Peanuts	Walnuts

Others:

Lean Lifestyle Guide -"KISS" Handout

Level 1 – The Basics – Do these 4 things over time & you will be in shape!

1. Just Move! Walk, walk, and walk some more. It doesn't have to be scheduled, but just make a point to walk more during the day. Park farther away, take more breaks at work, walk after lunch, etc.
2. Drink water! It doesn't get much simpler than that. Your body is 70% water, and you need more water if you want to burn body fat. Add lemon or cucumber for flavor. Swapping just ONE 12oz soda or fruit juice for water each day will save you 15 pounds over the course of a year! Shoot for 8 glasses, 80 ounces, and up to a gallon or more per day.
3. Small plates! Portion control is key. Eat your meals on salad plates, and use small bowls for cereals, soups, and desserts. Trick your mind. A "full" small plate looks better than the same food on a large plate with empty space.
4. Posture! Do the Lean Life Squeeze. Feet straight ahead, tighten your glutes (butt muscles), then your abs, and then pull your shoulders back, and stand tall with your head high. Hold it for 10 seconds to a minute or longer. Do it anytime anywhere. Nobody has to know!

Level 2 – The Next Steps – For those that want to get there faster.

- Eat 5 to 6 times per day. Have your 3 regular meals, and add a "mini-meal" (snack) between lunch & dinner and before bedtime. If you eat breakfast more than 5 hours before you eat lunch, eat a mini-meal mid-morning. Mini-meals should be about ½ to ¾ the size of the palm of your hand.
- Each meal should contain fats, carbohydrates, and protein. You want to avoid eating "just carbohydrates" for any snack or meal.

Level 3 – Dial it in! - You are ready to maximize your fat loss and get in top shape!

Build Your Meals - note: mini-meals should be about 1/3 the size of your main meals

Step 1 – Choose a lean protein from "Group 1" that is about the size of the palm of your hand.

Chicken, tuna, turkey, egg whites, low-fat cottage cheese, low-fat Greek yogurt, or lean red meat are good examples.

Step 2 – Add carbohydrates from "Group 2" (preferred) and/or "Group 3." If adding from Group 2, which are primarily fruits and vegetables, add DOUBLE the size of your protein portion (veggies – eat unlimited). If you are adding foods from Group 3, such as rice, grains, potatoes, bread, or pasta, which are generally higher-glycemic, make it the SAME size as the protein portion. If adding from both groups, decrease the Group 3 portion size by ½ or more.

- Group 2 - Fruits & veggies – most are great, so eat up! For Group 3, stick to whole grains & "brown" carbs. Minimize white grains, bread, rice, & pasta.

Step 3 – Add healthy fats that are about the size of your thumb. You want to consume poly & mono *unsaturated* fats, minimize saturated fats, and avoid all trans fats and hydrogenated oils.

- Best: almonds, avocado, olive/canola/grape seed/coconut oils, natural peanut butter, cashews, macadamia nuts, peanuts, omega-3 fish oils.
- Avoid/minimize: fatty red meats, egg yolks, organ meats like liver, shortenings, sour cream, cream cheese, cream, butter.

Step 4 – Time to eat! Start by eating some of your fats and protein. Fats will signal the brain to "stop eating" as well as slow the digestion of carbohydrates and insulin release into the system. The protein will trigger hormones that will further help to counteract the insulin release from the carbohydrates. That is why you want your fats and protein to reach your stomach first.

This is the natural way to keep your body burning fat while minimizing and eliminating cravings and the feeling you need to keep eating. Let your body work naturally, and you won't have to rely on willpower to stop eating.

Tips, tricks, and helpful hints

- Drink a glass of water about 20 minutes before every meal. This will help you burn fat, increase your metabolism, and will naturally help you eat less. Remember, a lot of "hunger" is just dehydration in disguise.
- This is easy; don't make it harder than it has to be. This guide can be loosely followed your entire life with great results. Always fall back on the basics: walk, water, portion control, and eat 5-6 times per day!
- Share with others in your community. It makes it easier if your family, friends, or co-workers are working towards the common goal of health along with you.

"Little things over time make a BIG difference when living the Lean Life!"

More info at: www.FitLife212.com

FitLife 212°

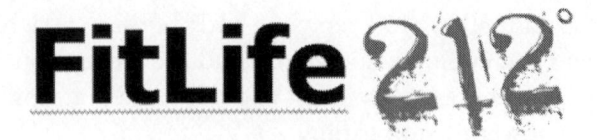

The Ten Commandments of a Lean Lifestyle

1. *Thou shall drink a minimum of 80 ounces of water a day*

2. *Thou shall look for opportunities to walk during the day*

3. *Thou shall eat a minimum of 5 times a day*

4. *Thou shall watch thy posture & thy portion sizes*

5. *Thou shall have protein & healthy fat at every meal*

6. *Thou shall strive to eat real food vs. processed food*

7. Thou must eliminate hydrogenated oils & corn syrup

8. Thou must exercise a minimum of 30 minutes per day

9. Thou must be positive & eliminate excuses

10. Thou must take responsibility for one's health & well being

Food Journal

Keep a log of everything you eat for a minimum of 3 days. Write down the time, what you ate (don't forget the "little" things like butter, sauces, creams, dressings, etc.), and make notes or comments on how the meal made you feel.

Time	What I Ate	Comments
Example: 8am	Bagel w/cream cheese	Hungry an hour later

About the Author

Brooks has a passion for health, fitness, and educating others dating back to his childhood. He began swimming competitively when he was six, was ranked 4th in the nation by the time he was ten, and went on to qualify for the Olympic Trials and NCAA's. He is a graduate of the United States Naval Academy, an entrepreneur, and a National Academy of Sports Medicine (NASM) Certified Personal Trainer and Corrective Exercise Specialist (CES). He has a passion and a commitment for educating people on the benefits of living a healthy lifestyle.

Email: *Brooks@FitLife212.com*

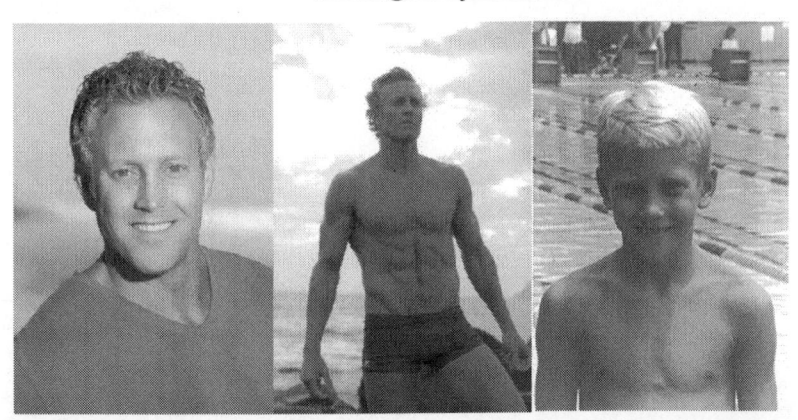

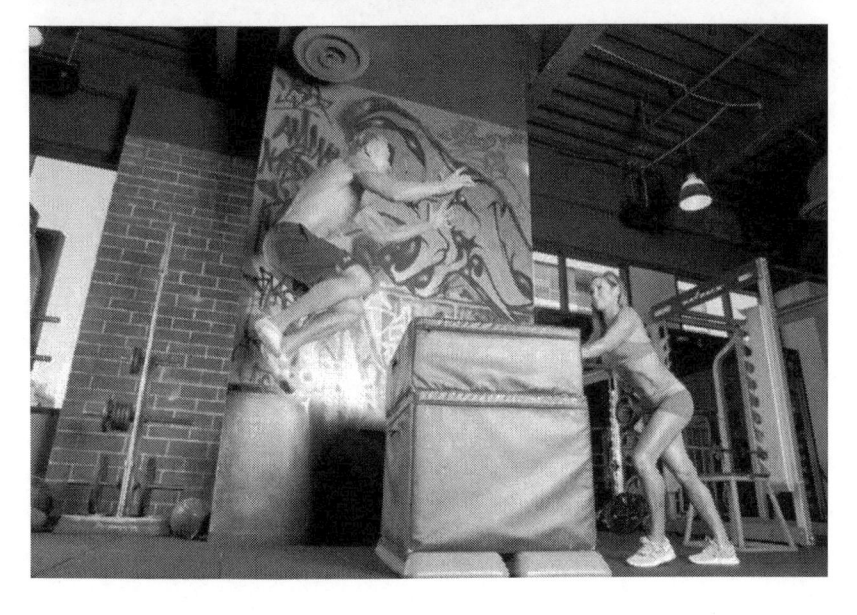

Printed in Great Britain
by Amazon.co.uk, Ltd.,
Marston Gate.